NEUROCHAOS

How COVID Rewired the Brains of Our Children

Dr. Katinka van der Merwe

Disclaimer

The information written in this book is designed to provide helpful information on pediatric long COVID and the subjects discussed. This book is not meant to be used to diagnose or treat any medical condition or to replace the advice of your physician(s). The author of this book does not claim to treat, diagnose, or cure pediatric long COVID or any other specific condition or infection. The author of this book treats the central nervous system only, often resulting in the body being able to heal itself.

The reader should regularly consult a physician in matters relating to his or her child's health, particularly with respect to any symptoms that may require diagnosis or medical attention. For diagnosis or treatment of any medical problem, consult your own physician(s).

The publisher and author are not responsible or liable for any damages or negative consequences from any treatment, action, application, or preparation to any person reading or following the information in this book. References are provided for informational purposes only and do not constitute endorsement of any websites or other sources. Readers should be aware that the websites listed in this book might change.

Table of Contents

My Story

Let me start with a question: what would you not do for your child?

If you're reading this, I imagine the answer is "nothing". There is nothing you wouldn't do to help your child heal, smile again, or simply feel like themselves. Whether your child has been battling Long COVID for weeks, months, or even years, I want you to know this: you are not alone, and there is still hope.

Every child is born with a purpose. I believe that with all my heart. Your child was not placed on this earth by accident, and their story is far from over. I don't know what brought you here—whether it was desperation, late-night Googling, or word-of-mouth from another parent—but I do know this. I've seen what happens when parents fight for their kids with everything they've got. I've seen transformations that defied every medical prediction. And I've seen kids go from barely getting out of bed to running, laughing, living again.

My own journey didn't begin in pediatrics or post-viral care. I was raised in Johannesburg, South Africa. My father was a chiropractor, and my mother embraced natural health like it was her calling.

Our home was grounded in a simple but powerful belief: the body is designed to heal. That philosophy shaped everything we did. We didn't reach for a prescription at the first sign of trouble. We supported the body, trusted its signals, and treated the cause—not just the symptoms.

That idea—that healing comes from within—has never left me. After we moved to the U.S., I followed in my father's footsteps, becoming a chiropractor and eventually joining his practice. But for years, I felt like something was missing.

I wanted more than to treat back and neck pain. I wanted to help people who had been told there were no answers. I wanted to reach the families who were falling through the cracks.

That clarity hit me hard when I met the father of two young patients. He had fallen from a ladder and shattered the vertebrae in his neck, leaving him paralyzed. I stood by his hospital bed, unable to help. I will never forget that feeling— helpless, heartbroken, and furious. That moment changed the course of my life. I promised myself I would never stop searching for answers again.

That promise led me to patients with complex regional pain syndrome (CRPS), Ehlers-Danlos Syndrome (EDS), and postural orthostatic tachycardia syndrome (POTS)—conditions that were often misunderstood and mismanaged. Many of these patients were children and teens. They were being dismissed, ignored, or overmedicated, often told it was "all in their head."

But I saw something different. I saw the root cause, and more importantly, I saw their potential to heal, even though conventional medicine declared EDS and CRPS to be "incurable".

Every week, patients from around the world entered our program and graduated in full remission in most cases. I did not let conventional medicine alter my belief system that fiercely held sacred the core belief that inborn intelligence leans to survival and healing, and it cannot be limited by words spoken by doctors, such as "incurable".

Then came Long COVID. At first, it showed up quietly—fatigue here, joint pain there, a child who couldn't keep up at school anymore. But soon, it became undeniable: we were facing something new, something complex. Children who had once been thriving were suddenly housebound. Some couldn't walk. Others couldn't eat.

Their bodies were failing them, and their parents were out of answers. These parents, out of sheer desperation, found us. Ayden was a very severe case, once featured in Time magazine. He was our pediatric long COVID "patient zero". His mom heard about our clinic and contacted us to see if we could help him.

My answer was honest. We do not know unless we try. In theory, we thought that the mechanism of injury by the COVID-19 virus was much the same as the patient population who developed severe and chronic systemic issues, as well as pain after viral infections. We weren't sure, but we felt optimistic. They decided to give our program a chance, and 15 weeks later, he left our program in full remission. Not only did our program work, but Long Covid was easier to treat than some of the other conditions we see. The thrill of helping that sweet boy recover after being so desperately disabled was powerful.

That's when I knew I had to act. I couldn't watch another child slip away while doctors told families to "wait it out." I began applying everything I had learned from treating complex neuroimmune disorders—only this time, I built a pediatric-focused program. It was gentler, more adaptable, and deeply individualized.

We reached other parents of severe long COVID patients as word of mouth grew. And it started working. And it worked again and again. We were even approached by a director of a pediatric long COVID program in Ohio, as we were helping some of their worst COVID patients, and word of mouth grew among parents of children in that program.

I've had the honor of helping children who hadn't left their beds in months walk out of my clinic. I've seen teens return to school, to sports, to laughter. And I've seen the fire come back into the eyes of parents who were once drowning in fear and guilt.

Out of these successes was born a genuine desire to help parents who are drowning in research and the desperation that stems from wanting to help one's own child. I wanted to share what was working for us and others in the circles in which I move.

This book was written for you. I wrote it for the parent searching for answers when the medical system says, "There's nothing else we can do." For the child who just wants to feel normal again. And for the families who refuse to give up— because I won't either.

It is absolutely essential that those working to help heal children with Long COVID come together—sharing their knowledge, resources, and real-world experience. Collaboration, not isolation, will move this field forward. We must openly exchange what is helping, what isn't, and what shows promise.

This spirit of shared discovery is the driving force behind this book: to equip you with practical tools, trusted resources, and above all, renewed hope. You are not alone in this fight, and neither is your child. You don't need blind faith to start this journey—just a willingness to see your child not as broken, but as full of potential.

Healing is possible. Hope is real. And I am honored to walk this road with you.

—Dr. Katinka

Chapter 1:
How Did You Get Here

"Believe in tomorrow. Hope will get you through today".

Unknown

"No storm, not even the one in your life, can last forever. The storm is just passing over."

Iyanla Vanzant

The Short History of Long COVID

There are moments in history that shift the world overnight—events that define generations. The moon landing. President John F. Kennedy's assassination. The 9/11 attacks. And then, there was SARS-CoV-2. Unlike a singular catastrophic event, COVID-19 unfolded in waves, creeping into every corner of life.

I remember the first moment I realized our world had changed. Schools were shutting down indefinitely. Parents, teachers, and students stood in confusion and fear. No one knew what was coming, yet in hindsight, the warning signs were everywhere. The tsunami had already begun.

COVID-19 took from us in ways both immediate and long-lasting—lives lost, economies shaken, relationships fractured. The global discourse became divisive, with debates raging over lockdowns, vaccines, and mandates. But this book is not about rehashing those battles. It is about what COVID left behind—a relentless storm of symptoms that refuses to fade.

The Origins of the Coronavirus Family

Coronaviruses have been around far longer than COVID-19. This family of viruses, first identified in the 1960s, includes strains responsible for illnesses ranging from the common cold to deadly respiratory syndromes like SARS and MERS. Named for the crown-like spikes on their surface, coronaviruses have a long history of jumping from animals to humans, evolving along the way.

The latest chapter of this history began on December 12, 2019, in Wuhan, China, when patients began exhibiting a mysterious pneumonia-like illness resistant to standard treatments. By the end of the month, the World Health Organization (WHO) was alerted. By January 3, 2020, China reported over 40 cases with an unknown cause. Just four days later, public health officials identified a novel coronavirus as the culprit. By January 20, the first confirmed U.S. case was reported, marking the beginning of a global crisis.

Since the onset of the COVID-19 pandemic, our understanding has evolved significantly. Today, many people question the initial narrative that the virus originated from a bat at a wet market in China. There is growing public concern that the origins of SARS-CoV-2, the virus behind COVID-19, may not be entirely natural.

Multiple U.S. government officials, including former CDC Director Dr. Robert Redfield, have publicly stated that the virus likely originated from a lab in Wuhan, China—a theory once dismissed but now considered plausible by the FBI and Department of Energy. In sworn congressional testimony, Dr. Anthony Fauci denied under oath that U.S. taxpayer funds were used to support gain-of-function research at the Wuhan Institute of Virology. Gain-of-function research is medical research that genetically alters an organism in a way that may enhance the biological functions of that organism.

However, NIH documents and independent reporting later revealed that grants funneled through EcoHealth Alliance may have supported risky research involving bat coronaviruses. Critics argue this presents a serious conflict of interest, especially given that Dr. Fauci's agency stood to benefit from vaccine development patents. While definitive proof remains under investigation, the ethical concerns surrounding transparency, scientific accountability, and financial gain during the pandemic rightfully continue to fuel debate.

As of this writing, over 7 million people have lost their lives to COVID-19. Entire decades of global health progress have been erased. Yet for many, COVID-19 is not just history—it is still their daily reality.

When COVID Doesn't End

For most individuals, COVID-19 is a temporary illness. Symptoms like fever, headache, cough, congestion, nausea, and fatigue appear and fade within a few weeks. But for a significant subset of people, particularly children, the virus doesn't seem to leave. This is where Long COVID enters the picture—an ongoing and debilitating condition that persists long after the initial infection has passed.

By definition, Long COVID, or post-acute sequelae of SARS-CoV-2 infection (PASC), refers to symptoms that last 12 weeks or longer following the initial COVID-19 infection. While many people recover relatively quickly, for others, the illness lingers, with symptoms waxing and waning or remaining constant over time. What makes Long COVID especially challenging is the sheer unpredictability of it. Not all individuals who contract COVID-19 go on to develop Long COVID, and we still don't fully understand why certain people, including children, are more susceptible than others. Some may experience only mild symptoms like fatigue or headaches, while others endure severe and debilitating conditions like difficulty breathing, chronic pain, or neurological dysfunction.

Unfortunately, the research landscape is fragmented and often inconsistent. Some studies rely on self-reported symptoms, making it difficult to draw reliable conclusions, while others are based on hospitalization data, which may not reflect the full scope of the population affected. The data we have is often biased, influenced by factors like geographic location, healthcare access, and vaccination status. As a result, it's challenging to form a comprehensive picture of Long COVID, especially in pediatric populations.

Despite the gaps in understanding, one thing is abundantly clear: Long COVID is not just a theoretical condition; it is a very real phenomenon that is wreaking havoc on children's lives. The impact of Long COVID on children goes beyond physical symptoms. It affects their ability to attend school, engage in extracurricular activities, and enjoy their normal childhood experiences. Parents are left to navigate an overwhelming maze of treatments, specialists, and therapies, often without clear guidance on what will help their child recover. Many pediatricians and specialists still underestimate or dismiss the gravity of Long COVID, which only adds to the burden faced by families seeking answers.

As we continue to learn more about Long COVID and its profound effects, it is crucial that we acknowledge the immense toll it takes, not only on the children directly affected but also on their families and communities. What we do know is this: Long COVID is real, and its consequences are far-reaching. Until we develop a deeper understanding of this condition, we must remain vigilant, advocate for those affected, and work together to find effective solutions that will restore the health and well-being of these young patients.

Rethinking the Word "Cure"

We often speak of a cure as something external—an intervention that eradicates illness from the outside in. But true healing is an internal process. The human body is designed to restore itself when given the right conditions. The nervous system plays a critical role in this process. While medications and therapies can support healing, they are not magic bullets. Misusing the word "cure" creates unrealistic expectations and undermines the body's intrinsic ability to recover.

When we hear the word *cure*, we often imagine a swift, external fix—a pill, a procedure, or a breakthrough treatment that wipes out illness and restores health overnight. But this view oversimplifies the complex, dynamic nature of true healing. A genuine return to health often begins not with something done *to* us, but with something awakened *within* us. The human body possesses remarkable innate intelligence—the capacity to repair, adapt, and even regenerate—when the right internal and external conditions are in place.

At the center of this self-healing system lies the nervous system, which serves as a master regulator of health. It communicates with every organ, modulates immune responses, governs inflammation, and interprets our environment. When the nervous system is dysregulated—through trauma, chronic stress, or illness—it can interrupt the body's healing signals, making recovery more difficult. Rebalancing and supporting the nervous system is therefore not just complementary to treatment; it's foundational.

While medications, supplements, and therapies can be powerful allies, they are not silver bullets. They can support the body, alleviate symptoms, and jumpstart biological processes, but they do not replace the body's inherent ability to heal. Misusing the word *cure*—especially in the context of complex, chronic illnesses like Long COVID, can create false hope or disillusionment. It may cause people to overlook or undervalue the slower, subtler, and more sustainable path of healing from the inside out.

A more accurate and empowering perspective is this: the role of medicine is not to *cure* in the traditional sense, but to *facilitate the conditions in which healing can occur*. When we shift from seeking a cure to cultivating healing, we open the door to more compassionate, patient-centered care—especially for children whose bodies are still growing and adapting in response to illness.

The Shortcomings of Modern Medicine

Pediatric Long COVID has illuminated deep cracks in the foundation of modern healthcare—cracks that families now face firsthand. While parents search desperately for answers, many encounter a medical system that is reactive rather than proactive, fragmented rather than unified.

- **Symptom Management Over Root Cause Treatment:** In conventional medicine, the emphasis is placed on suppressing symptoms instead of identifying and correcting the root dysfunction. Fatigue is treated with stimulants, pain with analgesics, and anxiety with sedatives—yet none of these strategies address *why* the symptoms exist in the first place. For children with Long COVID, this surface-level approach often leads to a

frustrating cycle of temporary relief and recurring
illness.

• **Pharmaceutical Dependence:** The default
answer in many medical settings is a prescription pad.
While medications can provide short-term help, they
rarely offer long-term healing—and every drug carries
the risk of side effects, some of which can further
destabilize an already fragile system. Children are left
navigating a cocktail of medications with no cohesive
plan to restore true health.

• **Siloed Specialists:** Families are often bounced
between pulmonologists, neurologists, cardiologists,
gastroenterologists, and infectious disease experts—each
operating within their own narrowly defined specialty.
While these professionals may be well-meaning, they
rarely communicate or coordinate care, and too often
miss the bigger picture. As a result, connections between
symptoms go unrecognized, and opportunities for
integrated healing are lost.

• **Lack of a Holistic Approach:** Western medicine
tends to treat the body as a collection of isolated parts.
But children are not machines with faulty components
to replace; they are dynamic, interconnected systems.
When Long COVID disrupts that system, healing must
involve the whole child—body, brain, and
environment—not just a single organ or symptom.

• **Failure to Recognize Nervous System
Involvement:** Perhaps one of the most glaring
omissions in conventional care is the failure to address
the role of the autonomic nervous system. Long COVID

often leads to dysautonomia, neuroinflammation, and imbalanced immune signaling—yet these central regulators are rarely acknowledged, let alone treated. Ignoring the nervous system means overlooking one of the primary levers for healing.

Pediatric Long COVID has exposed what many integrative and functional practitioners have long known: our current medical model is not designed for chronic, complex, systemic illness. It excels at crisis care—broken bones, infections, surgeries—but falls short when the healing requires nuance, time, and a systems-based approach. Until we shift toward whole-child, root-cause medicine, children with Long COVID will continue to suffer in a system not built to understand them.

Pediatric Post-COVID Care Centers (PCCCs) are emerging to fill this gap, offering rehabilitation-focused treatment. However, these centers are overwhelmed with long waitlists, inconsistent results, and limited holistic options. Children with neurological symptoms often fare the worst.

Who is Most at Risk for Pediatric Long COVID?

While any child can develop Long COVID, risk factors include:

- Severity of Initial Infection – More severe cases may lead to prolonged symptoms, though even mild cases can result in Long COVID.

- Age – Older children may report symptoms more clearly than younger ones, skewing data.

- Gender – While both boys and girls are affected, our experience shows more boys seeking treatment for severe cases.

- Pre-Existing Conditions – Chronic illnesses, metabolic disorders, genetic disorders, autoimmune diseases, hypermobility spectrum issues, and sleep disturbances increase risk.

I want to especially expand on the link between Long COVID and hypermobility disorders. Emerging research indicates that children with hypermobile Ehlers-Danlos syndrome (hEDS) or hypermobility spectrum disorders (HSD) may be at increased risk for developing Long COVID. A study published in *BMJ Public Health* found that individuals with generalized joint hypermobility were 30% more likely to experience prolonged symptoms after COVID-19 infection, including persistent fatigue—a hallmark of Long COVID (1). We are seeing that *almost every patient* with Long COVID also has hypermobility, most often undiagnosed. What complicates this is that the criteria for diagnosing hEDS and HSD is outdated and sometimes outright incorrect. For example, many patients with hEDS or HSD ironically do NOT have hypermobile joints. Importantly, hEDS and HSD are not solely defined by visible joint hypermobility. Many patients, especially children, may not exhibit overt hyperflexibility but still suffer from underlying connective tissue abnormalities that affect multiple systems, including the autonomic nervous system. This can lead to symptoms such as dizziness, rapid heartbeat, and gastrointestinal issues, which are also common in Long COVID.

In practice, we are noticing an explosion of hEDS and HSD post-COVID and post-COVID vaccine. I believe that while this disorder is not always expressed genetically, it can become expressed (or symptomatic) by illness, trauma, or vaccines.

The overlap in symptoms suggests a shared pathophysiology between hEDS/HSD and Long COVID, potentially involving immune dysregulation and autonomic nervous system dysfunction. Recognizing this connection is crucial for healthcare providers to identify at-risk pediatric patients and tailor management strategies accordingly.

Emerging research is uncovering biomarkers associated with Long COVID. A 2023 study identified distinct immune and hormonal differences in Long COVID patients, including low cortisol levels, abnormal T-cell activity, and Epstein-Barr virus reactivation. These findings may pave the way for targeted treatment strategies (2).

Why Pediatric Long COVID is Being Neglected

Research on pediatric Long COVID remains scarce because children were not the primary focus during the initial phases of the pandemic. Funding priorities have leaned toward adult cases and vaccine development, leaving pediatric research underfunded and deprioritized. Additionally, because children often recover quickly from acute infections, long-term effects have been underestimated. Many healthcare institutions lack standardized guidelines for diagnosing and treating pediatric Long COVID, further discouraging large-scale studies. Without strong advocacy and dedicated funding, the medical community continues to overlook the urgent need for pediatric-focused research.

Studies estimate that anywhere from 5% to 40% of children experience lingering symptoms post-infection (3). Children also struggle to articulate their symptoms, making diagnosis difficult. Parents may notice appetite loss, fatigue, or mood changes without realizing their child is battling Long COVID. Pediatric Long COVID has been largely neglected due to a combination of factors. First, children were initially believed to be less affected by the virus, leading to minimal research and delayed recognition of long-term consequences. Second, because children may struggle to articulate their symptoms, their conditions are often dismissed or misdiagnosed. Additionally, research funding has primarily focused on adult Long COVID cases, leaving pediatric cases underrepresented. Finally, the medical system's emphasis on acute care rather than long-term recovery means many healthcare providers lack awareness or structured treatment plans for affected children. As a result, countless children suffering from Long COVID are left without the support and care they desperately need.

Testing for Long COVID

Diagnosing pediatric Long COVID is an uphill battle because there is no single test that can definitively confirm it. Instead, doctors rely on a patchwork of evaluations—blood work, inflammatory markers, imaging scans, and autonomic function tests—to piece together a diagnosis. But here's the frustrating reality: these tests often come back "normal," leaving both parents and doctors without clear answers. Meanwhile, children continue to struggle with debilitating symptoms like relentless fatigue, brain fog, chronic pain, and nervous system dysfunction—symptoms that don't always show up on standard medical tests. This lack of clear diagnostic criteria means too many children are left undiagnosed, misunderstood, and without the care they desperately need. For families, this often leads to an exhausting cycle of searching for answers, advocating for their child, and pushing the medical system to recognize what they are going through. The bottom line? Pediatric Long COVID is real, and these children deserve better.

Thoughts on the COVID vaccine for children

When I started this book, I was highly conflicted about what I would and would not say about the COVID-19 vaccine for children. The world is still not a safe place when it comes to openly expressing one's negative thoughts on this vaccine for children. I have personally seen the actual damage that this vaccine can cause. I maintain that some of the side effects caused by it will only become known in the future. My husband and I chose not to vaccinate our children for COVID-19. We ourselves also did not get vaccinated. Every parent must make their own decision for their child, and that decision, at the very least, should be an educated one. I believe that the decision to vaccinate or not vaccinate one's child should come down to a simple risk-benefit analysis.

The risk-benefit profile of the COVID-19 vaccine for healthy children remains highly controversial and, for many, simply does not justify widespread use. The data clearly show that healthy children have an extremely low risk of severe outcomes from COVID-19. According to CDC data, the infection fatality rate for children under 18 is estimated to be between 0.001% and 0.01%, depending on age and underlying health conditions. A large UK study published in *Nature* found that the absolute risk of death from COVID-19 in children was two per million—a statistically negligible figure (4). Conversely, emerging evidence suggests that certain groups, especially those with connective tissue disorders like undiagnosed hypermobility spectrum disorders or Ehlers-Danlos Syndrome, may be more susceptible to adverse effects from vaccines, particularly those affecting autonomic and cardiovascular regulation.

A 2023 peer-reviewed study in *Frontiers in Pharmacology* noted that up to 87% of patients with hypermobility-related disorders experienced post-vaccine symptom flare-ups, including dysautonomia, POTS, and neuropathic pain (5). Furthermore, cases of myocarditis and pericarditis, particularly in adolescent males, have been consistently reported following mRNA vaccination, sometimes requiring hospitalization. These risks are not just theoretical. The FDA's own briefing documents acknowledge the increased risk of myocarditis in children post-vaccine and have approved the pediatric vaccines under Emergency Use Authorization rather than full approval, despite limited long-term safety data.

Critics argue that the one-size-fits-all public health messaging ignores biologically vulnerable subgroups and fails to account for individual risk tolerance. Given the low threat COVID poses to healthy children and the increasing reports of post-vaccine complications—even if rare—the precautionary principle supports a more cautious, individualized approach, especially when natural infection in children generally results in mild illness and robust immunity.

Fear is a powerful motivator, however. What if you are terrified that your child will get COVID again? The majority of cases that we have treated with long COVID did get the vaccine, although some patients didn't. In the cases that we have treated, the vaccine did not prevent Long COVID. Several studies have shown that COVID-19 vaccines do not reliably prevent Long COVID, particularly in younger or low-risk populations. A large study published in *Nature Medicine* (Al-Aly et al., 2022) found that while vaccination modestly reduced the

risk of developing Long COVID (by about 15%), it did not
eliminate the risk, and many vaccinated individuals still
experienced persistent symptoms after breakthrough infections
(6).

Another UK-based study in *The Lancet Respiratory
Medicine* (2022) found that vaccinated individuals who became
infected had only a slightly lower incidence of Long COVID
compared to unvaccinated individuals—suggesting that
vaccination offers limited protection against post-viral
complications (7). This aligns with emerging data indicating
that immune dysregulation and viral persistence, not just
severity of acute illness, contribute to Long COVID—factors
that are not fully mitigated by vaccination.

A new study published in 2025 found that the spike protein
is detected in 92% of vaccine-injured patients up to 245 days
after the injection, raising serious concerns about post-
vaccination chronic disease. It further studied post-vaccine
chronic illnesses and found that the overlap in symptoms
implies that immune responses to SARS-CoV-2 (or its
components)—*whether via infection or vaccination*—can trigger
prolonged immune activation in vulnerable individuals,
including children (8). It is possible that the very thing that you
hope will protect your child from future COVID infections- the
vaccine- may cause the same awful injuries

The decision to vaccinate or not vaccinate a child with
Long COVID can be an agonizing one. After all, you have
personally seen what this virus can do. I understand your fear.
However, I am here to tell you that vaccinating your child will
not necessarily protect him or her. In fact, it can make things
much worse. Emerging evidence and clinical observations
suggest that children already suffering from Long COVID may

be at increased risk of adverse reactions following COVID-19 vaccination. A study published in *Nature Immunology* (2023) noted that individuals with ongoing post-viral syndromes, including Long COVID, often display immune dysregulation and persistent inflammation, which may heighten their vulnerability to vaccine-related side effects due to a hyper-responsive or exhausted immune system (9).

Though large-scale pediatric-specific data are still limited, many clinicians and researchers urge caution and call for individualized risk-benefit analysis before administering additional doses to children already experiencing complex post-viral syndromes.

This is a complicated issue, and I certainly understand that. For me? Given everything I know? I'd rather not.

What is a spike protein?

The spike protein is a structural component found on the surface of the SARS-CoV-2 virus—the virus responsible for COVID-19. It is this protein that allows the virus to attach to and enter human cells by binding to the ACE2 receptors, which are found in the lungs, heart, brain, and many other tissues. This interaction is central to how the virus infects the body. Research has shown that the spike protein alone, even without the rest of the virus, can cause inflammation, damage to endothelial cells, and disruption of vascular integrity (10).

This may help explain why some children experience ongoing symptoms after COVID-19, as lingering spike proteins or spike-induced immune reactions may continue to affect sensitive systems like the nervous and cardiovascular systems. Understanding the spike protein's role is essential in unraveling the mechanisms behind pediatric long COVID and developing effective treatments.

Concerns have been raised about the potential for vaccine-induced spike protein to be shed and affect others. Studies have detected circulating spike protein in the blood of individuals who developed myocarditis after mRNA vaccination. A study published in *Circulation* found that adolescents with post-vaccine myocarditis had markedly higher levels of free full-length spike protein in their plasma compared to asymptomatic vaccinated individuals, suggesting a potential link between spike protein presence and adverse events (11).

Furthermore, research has indicated that the spike protein and vaccine mRNA may persist in the body longer than initially anticipated. A study in *Pharmacological Research Perspectives* reported that modified SARS-CoV-2 mRNA could persist up to a month post-injection, with recombinant spike protein detectable in the blood for over six months (12).

While spike protein shedding remains a poorly understood phenomenon, emerging evidence raises a sobering possibility: that the very vaccine intended to protect against COVID-19 may, in rare cases, contribute to the same types of debilitating outcomes it aims to prevent. This unsettling parallel warrants deeper inquiry, not dismissal.

What is Spike Protein Shedding After Vaccination?

Spike protein shedding refers to the theoretical or suspected release of SARS-CoV-2 spike protein (produced in response to mRNA or adenoviral vector COVID-19 vaccines) into extracellular spaces, body fluids, or even potentially from one person to another. This is distinct from viral shedding and does not involve infectious virus.

COVID-19 vaccines like Pfizer-BioNTech and Moderna use mRNA technology to instruct cells to produce the SARS-CoV-2 spike protein, which then stimulates an immune response. Some concerns—particularly among vaccine-injured communities—have been raised about:

- Whether circulating spike protein persists longer than intended, whether this contributes to post-vaccine illness, and whether the spike protein could be excreted or "shed" from vaccinated individuals.

At least one study has revealed that the spike protein can persist far longer than anticipated following vaccination, with detectable levels found in lymphatic tissue for up to two months. This extended presence challenges earlier assumptions about how quickly the body clears vaccine-derived proteins and invites further investigation into potential long-term effects (13).

The Future of Treatment

Research is slowly beginning to shift focus toward pediatric-specific solutions. The NIH's RECOVER Initiative is leading efforts to understand how Long COVID impacts children, while global clinical trials are exploring potential interventions. However, funding remains inadequate. The healthcare system still prioritizes preventing severe acute COVID over addressing Long COVID's long-term effects.

Certain biomarkers may soon help match patients to targeted treatments (14). *In addition,* holistic approaches—combining nervous system rehabilitation, immune support, and metabolic therapies—are showing promise (15), as will become abundantly evident as you read this book.

While much remains unknown, one fact is clear: the battle against Long COVID is far from over. But with knowledge comes power, and with power comes change. It is time to fight for the children left behind in this pandemic's wake. They are not without hope, as this book can attest.

Chapter 2:
Common Symptoms

"Loneliness is the feeling of being alone even when you're surrounded by people."

Wayne Dyer

"It's so hard to pretend to be okay when it feels like the whole world is crumbling around you."

Last of the Lancers

Children with Long COVID often feel misunderstood, isolated, and dismissed. They are battling a condition that is not only new but also complex, making it difficult for them to articulate what they are experiencing. Their symptoms are vast, unpredictable, and frequently misunderstood—even by medical professionals. This uncertainty extends to their families, who struggle to find clear answers and effective treatment in a healthcare system that has yet to fully grasp the condition's scope.

Despite the mounting evidence, Long COVID remains a puzzle for doctors and researchers. Many families are left to become their own detectives, piecing together symptoms, researching tirelessly, and seeking support from others facing the same challenges. They are forced into advocacy roles they never expected, simply to ensure their child is heard, validated, and treated.

Taking control of your child's health is a **powerful** step. It transforms you from a bystander into an active participant, arming you with knowledge and the ability to fight for the care your child deserves. Understanding the symptoms is the first step—because when you know what you're dealing with, you can take action. Your child's illness is real. It is not in their head. And you are not alone in this battle.

Pediatric Long COVID presents an overwhelming range of symptoms. Some children may experience just one or two lingering effects, while others suffer from an extensive, debilitating list. To further complicate matters, many of these symptoms overlap with other medical conditions, making diagnosis and treatment even more challenging. The severity of the initial infection offers no clear predictor of whether a child will develop Long COVID—cases have been documented in children who had severe, mild, or even asymptomatic COVID-19 infections.

Additionally, a growing number of children with Long COVID develop secondary conditions, further blurring the lines between cause and effect. These secondary illnesses can range from chronic fatigue syndrome and postural orthostatic tachycardia syndrome (POTS) to autoimmune disorders and neurological complications. The return of symptoms, or symptom flare-ups, may be triggered by new infections, physical or emotional stress, or in some cases, with no clear cause at all.

At this time, there is **no single test** that definitively diagnoses pediatric Long COVID. Diagnosis is a process of elimination—ruling out other conditions with overlapping symptoms. Unfortunately, most pediatricians are not yet trained to recognize or diagnose Long COVID in children, leaving many young patients undiagnosed or misdiagnosed.

Many other conditions share symptoms with Long COVID, including chronic fatigue syndrome, fibromyalgia, mast cell activation syndrome (MCAS), amplified musculoskeletal pain syndrome (AMPS), and myalgic encephalomyelitis.

Additionally, children with pre-existing conditions such as type 2 diabetes, Ehlers-Danlos Syndrome (EDS), asthma, lung disease, heart failure, obesity, and autoimmune diseases may be at greater risk of developing Long COVID.

COVID-19 is not just a respiratory virus—it is a **multi-system disease** that can cause long-term damage to the heart, lungs, brain, liver, kidneys, and nervous system. It increases the risk of developing or worsening medical conditions, including POTS, diabetes, kidney disease, and chronic neurological pain. The symptoms reported in pediatric Long COVID cases vary widely in severity—some children are able to maintain their daily routines, while others are completely debilitated, unable to participate in normal life.

The fight for answers continues, but one thing is clear: Long COVID is real, and its impact on children is profound. Parents must take an active role in advocating for their child's health, arming themselves with information, seeking out knowledgeable healthcare providers, and refusing to accept dismissive responses. **Your child's suffering is real, and they deserve to be heard, understood, and treated.**

Whole body:

- Abnormal movements
- Allodynia (skin sensitivity, especially sensitivity to light touch)
- Amplified pain syndrome (AMPS)
- Autoimmune diseases such as rheumatoid arthritis and lupus
- Back pain

- Burning pain

- Chronic inflammation

- Decreased immune function

- Deep aching "bone-crushing" pain

- Diabetes

- Dysautonomia

- Extreme fatigue/tiredness/lack of energy that interferes with daily life

- Fever and chills

- Functional neurologic disorder (FND)

- Mast cell activation syndrome (MCAS)

- Multisystem inflammatory disorder (MID-C)

- Neurologic pain

- Repeated viral and/or bacterial infections

- Sleep problems, including insomnia, extreme daytime sleepiness, and restless leg syndrome

- Symptoms that worsen after physical or mental activity (post-exertional malaise)

- Weakness

Brain/Nerves:

- Brain fog/difficulty concentrating, remembering, or focusing (described as feeling "separated from the world")

- Functional Neurologic Disorder (FND)

- Headaches

- Lightheadedness and/or dizziness upon standing/vertigo
- Memory loss
- Mental health conditions such as anxiety or depression
- Mood changes
- Moodiness
- Neurological tremors
- Obsessive-Compulsive Disorder (OCD)
- Phobias/fear of specific things
- Post-Traumatic Stress Disorder (PTSD)
- Seizures/tremors/non-epileptic seizures
- Sleep disorders
- Thoughts of hopelessness and even suicide
- Tics (verbal and other)
- Tingling, numbness, and nerve damage

Eyes:

- Blurry vision
- Hypersensitivity to light
- Inability to focus eyes
- Loss of visual acuity

Ears:

- Dizziness or vertigo
- Ear pain or pressure
- Hearing loss

- Tinnitus (ringing in the ears)

Smell/Taste:

- Stuffy nose

- Loss of taste or a distorted sense of taste

- Loss of smell or a distorted sense of smell

Neck/Throat:

- Choking sensation

- Difficulty swallowing (dysphagia)

- Dry mouth or throat irritation

- Eosinophilic esophagitis

- Hoarseness

- Lump in the throat sensation

- Neck pain

- Sore throat

- Tightness in the throat

Lungs:

- Breathing difficulty
- Cough
- Shortness of breath and/or difficulty breathing
- Wheezing

Heart and Blood:

- Chest Pain
- Rapid or irregular heartbeat
- Fainting
- Blood clots/microclots, and blood vessel issues

Kidneys/Bladder:

- Changes in urination
- Interstitial cystitis (IC)
- New or worsening overactive bladder (known as Covid-19
- associated cystitis (CAC)

Hands:

- Raynaud's syndrome

Legs/Feet:

- Swelling in the legs or feet
- Raynaud's syndrome

Reproductive Systems:

- Changes in the menstrual cycle
- Female infertility

- Long-term decline of ovarian health, including premature ovarian insufficiency (POI)

- Reduced male fertility

- Worsening premenstrual symptoms

- Complicated menstrual cycles that may include a combination of symptoms ramping up after ovulation and before menstruation. These may include nerve pain, brain fog, migraines, and facial pain, to name a few

There is also a chance that in the future, Long Covid could lead to what is commonly seen in adults with Long Covid:

- Possibility of a higher risk of preeclampsia

- Possibility of a higher risk of preterm birth

Digestive Systems:

- Loss of appetite

- Stomach pain

- Changes in appetite

- Diarrhea

- Heartburn

- Changes in stool color

- Nausea

- Vomiting

- Bloating

- Gluten intolerance/allergies

- Gastroparesis

- Food intolerances

Skin/Hair:

- Rashes

- Hair loss

- Skin color changes (e.g, red, white, or purple skin color changes)

Muscles and bones:

- Muscle aches

- Joint pain

- Reduced mobility

If you don't see your child's specific symptom on this list, don't lose hope. Long COVID is still being studied, and new discoveries are emerging. The lack of recognition today does not mean your child's experience isn't real. Your role as an advocate is critical—seeking answers, connecting with others, and refusing to accept dismissal can make all the difference.

Knowledge is power, and your voice matters. The more parents, patients, and medical professionals speak up, the more awareness and research will follow. Your child's diagnosis is not a sentence—it's a starting point. What you believe about their recovery shapes their reality. Who is responsible for their health? You are. Who cares most about their well-being? You do. That means taking charge, questioning everything, and ensuring no stone is left unturned.

I hope this chapter brings clarity and reassurance. If you recognize your child's struggles in these pages, know you are not alone. Understanding their symptoms is the first step toward real progress. If new or alarming symptoms arise, don't hesitate to seek medical advice. Long COVID is complex, but it should never be an excuse to overlook other potential conditions.

Never let a doctor—or anyone—dismiss your concerns. Trust your instincts. Stay vigilant. Your child's health is in your hands, and with that comes both responsibility and empowerment. Stay relentless in your pursuit of answers, because your child deserves nothing less.

Chapter 3:
Secondary Conditions Associated With Long Covid

"Out of suffering have emerged the strongest souls; the most massive characters are seared with scars."

Kahlil Gibran

"Courage doesn't always roar. Sometimes courage is the quiet voice at the end of the day saying, 'I will try again tomorrow.'"

Mary Anne Radmacher

After a child experiences Long COVID, it's possible for secondary conditions to develop—these are new health issues that arise as a result of the stress or damage caused by the original illness. These are not just lingering symptoms of COVID itself, but entirely separate diagnoses that emerge *after* the body has been fighting the virus for some time. For example, a child who seemed to be slowly recovering might suddenly develop Functional Neurological Disorder (FND), where the brain has trouble sending and receiving signals properly, leading to movement difficulties, fainting, or other nervous system problems. Others may develop POTS (Postural Orthostatic Tachycardia Syndrome), a condition affecting heart rate and blood flow, or even autoimmune disorders where the immune system begins attacking the body's own tissues. These conditions can be confusing and scary for families, especially if they appear to come "out of nowhere." But understanding them as secondary conditions—triggered by the original COVID infection—can help guide families toward more targeted treatments and reassure them that their child's experience is real, known, and treatable.

In conventional medicine, when new symptoms arise, they're often given new names—new diagnoses that come with separate treatments, specialists, and medications. But this way of thinking can be misleading, especially when it comes to pediatric Long COVID. Just because a child develops additional symptoms over time doesn't mean they've developed a completely new illness. It means the original problem—the impact of the virus on their body—is still unfolding. Instead of chasing each symptom with a different label or treatment, we must step back and see the whole picture. These aren't separate conditions; they're part of the same story. The real solution isn't to keep changing the diagnosis—it's to heal the underlying damage. When we treat the root cause and support the body as a whole, symptoms begin to resolve. Healing doesn't come from managing labels. It comes from restoring balance at the source.

Your approach has to be as follows: "We have this new diagnosis now, but it's not an additional condition to figure out and manage, it is just another group of symptoms, caused by the same thing. The damage the virus caused is the problem. The fact that my child's body was unusually vulnerable to this damage when other kids skate by, THAT is the problem. That's where you have to start.

Listed below, you will find the conditions that we are noticing post Long COVID in the field, working with real-life Long COVID patients.

Several secondary conditions have been documented in pediatric patients following COVID-19 infection, both in clinical studies and through patient reports on social media. These conditions, distinct from the initial symptoms of COVID-19, may emerge weeks or months after the acute phase of the illness. Below is a list of such conditions with supporting evidence:

Amplified Musculoskeletal Pain Syndrome (AMPS)

AMPS is a condition where children experience chronic pain in their muscles, joints, or other parts of the body without any clear injury or inflammation. This pain can be constant or come and go, and it might affect the whole body or just one area. Children with AMPS may also have heightened sensitivity to touch, temperature, or movement, making everyday activities challenging. Their bodies become like exposed, live nerves, easily triggered by (for example) flowing water touching the skin, clothing, the smallest wisp of air, vibration, noise, or temperature fluctuation. Increased atmospheric pressure may increase their pain, as well as the stress of any kind. Their pain is invisible and often thought to be psychogenic or not "real". It is real.

After recovering from COVID-19, some children develop AMPS as part of their long COVID symptoms. The virus may disrupt the way the nervous system processes pain, leading to an overactive pain response. This means that the nerves send stronger pain signals than they should, even without a physical cause. This condition is more common in adolescent girls, but it can affect any child.

Diagnosing AMPS involves ruling out other conditions through medical history, physical exams, and sometimes tests like blood work or imaging. Since there are no specific tests for AMPS, it's essential for healthcare providers to recognize the symptoms and understand the child's experience.

Common Signs of Pediatric AMPS in Pediatric Long COVID:

- Persistent, severe pain out of proportion to any injury

- Pain that moves or spreads to other areas of the body

- Allodynia (pain from normally non-painful stimuli, like light touch or clothing)

- Changes in skin temperature or color in the painful area (red, purple, or pale)

- Swelling in the affected limb

- Joint stiffness or reduced mobility

- Muscle weakness in the affected area

- Fatigue and poor sleep due to pain

- Avoidance of using the painful limb (limping or guarding)

- Anxiety or stress associated with the pain

- School refusal or difficulty participating in normal activities

- History of a minor illness or injury before symptoms began

We have noticed that AMPS is a common condition in Long COVID pediatric patients. It is also one of the conditions that causes children with Long COVID the most pain. There is emerging evidence suggesting that Amplified Musculoskeletal Pain Syndrome (AMPS) may develop in pediatric patients following COVID-19 infections, including those with Long COVID. AMPS is characterized by chronic pain in muscles and joints without any clear injury or inflammation. In children, this condition can lead to widespread pain, sensitivity to touch, and other symptoms such as headaches and fatigue.

A study published in the *Journal of PLOS Digital Health* identified a subphenotype of pediatric Long COVID characterized by musculoskeletal pain, affecting 13.9% of the cohort. These findings suggest that AMPS may be a secondary condition that arises after a COVID-19 infection, particularly in children who experience persistent pain and other related symptoms. The study utilized electronic health record data to identify distinct clinical presentations, or subphenotypes, of Long COVID in children. The study found that musculoskeletal pain was a significant component in one of these subphenotypes, affecting approximately 13.9% of the pediatric cohort (1).

Early recognition and appropriate management are crucial to help affected children recover and improve their quality of life.

Anxiety

Many children recovering from COVID-19 are facing a new challenge they didn't have before: persistent anxiety. This isn't just typical childhood worry—it's often intense, unpredictable, and physically distressing. Studies have shown that anxiety is one of the most commonly reported symptoms in children with Long COVID, affecting both their emotional well-being and ability to participate in daily activities like school, play, and social interaction. In fact, research from the RECOVER pediatric cohort identified anxiety and mood symptoms as part of a key subphenotype of Long COVID in children (2).

This kind of anxiety often appears alongside other symptoms like fatigue, sleep disturbances, or even chest pain, making it hard to spot as a separate issue. Parents may notice their child becoming more irritable, withdrawn, or overwhelmed by small challenges. It's important to understand that this anxiety is not "just in their head"—it's part of a larger physiological disruption triggered by the virus's impact on the nervous system, interestingly enough.

Research indicates that children with a history of anxiety are more susceptible to developing long COVID symptoms, including heightened anxiety levels (3). This is a significant clue. Anxiety is most often a sign of autonomic nervous system dysfunction. This finding supports the premise that nervous system dysfunction most likely *precedes* Long COVID, as discussed in this book.

Complex Regional Pain Syndrome (CRPS)

Complex Regional Pain Syndrome (CRPS) is a chronic and often misunderstood pain condition that can develop after even a minor injury, illness, or medical event. In CRPS, the nervous system becomes overly sensitive and misfires, sending constant pain signals to the brain—even when there is no actual threat or injury present. It's like the body's pain alarm gets stuck in the "on" position and can't shut off. The nervous system of children and adults with CRPS becomes overly sensitive, causing long-lasting pain, swelling, and other symptoms—even after the original injury has healed. In patients with severe COVID-19, nerve damage can happen for several reasons, like inflammation caused by the virus, the way the patient was positioned while being treated, or as a side effect of medical procedures.

While scientists don't yet fully understand how COVID-19 may cause this kind of pain, they believe that the intense inflammation that happens during a severe infection may overwhelm the nervous system and make it more likely to develop CRPS.

In children, CRPS often starts in one limb—such as an arm, leg, hand, or foot—and may involve symptoms like intense burning pain, swelling, changes in skin color or temperature, sensitivity to touch or movement, and even muscle weakness or stiffness. Over time, and especially if untreated, the pain and other symptoms can spread to nearby areas or even to the opposite side of the body.

This condition can deeply affect a child's ability to move, play, or go to school. CRPS isn't just "in their head"—it's a real disorder of the nervous system. While it can be extremely painful and frightening, early recognition and treatment—especially approaches that calm the nervous system—can make a significant difference in a child's recovery.

Common Symptoms of CRPS in Pediatric Long COVID:

- Continuous, burning, or throbbing pain (usually in an arm, leg, hand, or foot)

- Sensitivity to touch or cold (allodynia)

- Swelling in the affected area

- Changes in skin temperature (alternating between sweaty and cold)

- Changes in skin color (pale, blotchy, red, purple, or blue)

- Changes in skin texture (shiny, thin, or excessively sweaty skin)

- Joint stiffness and swelling

- Muscle weakness and atrophy (wasting)

- Decreased range of motion

- Abnormal hair and nail growth in the affected limb

- Pain that spreads beyond the initial area of injury

Several case studies have documented the onset of CRPS after COVID-19 infection. For instance, a case study described a patient who developed CRPS type 1 following a COVID-19 infection, suggesting a potential link between the virus and the development of CRPS (4). Another report detailed a case of CRPS in a patient after severe COVID-19, highlighting the potential neurological complications associated with the virus (5). Although there are no studies yet about the link between Long COVID and CRPS, we have treated several pediatric patients who developed CRPS shortly after a COVID-19 infection. It is therefore my belief that COVID is a definite risk factor for CRPS.

The exact mechanism by which COVID-19 may lead to CRPS is not fully understood, but it is hypothesized that the virus's impact on the nervous system and immune response could play a role. These findings underscore the importance of monitoring for chronic pain conditions like CRPS in patients recovering from COVID-19.

CRPS is easier to treat early. Therefore, it is crucial to obtain a correct diagnosis as soon as possible. Sadly, because CRPS is so rare and misunderstood, many doctors will misdiagnose it or miss it altogether. It can sometimes present with tell-tale signs, such as loss of hair, shiny skin, discoloration, swelling, and even blisters and scabs. However, sometimes it can present without physical signs. Children, especially, may face an uphill battle in being believed by their healthcare team. Please familiarize yourself with the early signs and symptoms of this condition, which usually (but not always) develop after surgeries or injuries. In order to protect your child, be aware of the following:

- **Vagus nerve stimulation** is very important to protect a child against the development of CRPS. If your child is going to undergo surgery, including oral surgery, stimulate the vagus nerve for up to four weeks prior to the procedure. Use a Rezzimax© for best results (described in chapter 7).

- Studies have shown that **vitamin C supplementation** can decrease the risk of developing CRPS after wrist fractures and other extremity injuries (6). In children, the use of vitamin C to prevent Complex Regional Pain Syndrome (CRPS) after surgery or trauma is not as well-studied as in adults, but careful adaptation from adult protocols can be considered. In adults, the standard preventive dose is 500 mg of vitamin C daily for 50 days. For children, the 50-day daily dose should be adjusted based on age and weight, keeping in mind the tolerable upper intake levels (ULs) recommended by the Institute of Medicine. For example, children ages 4 to 8 can safely take 250 to 400 mg daily, those 9 to 13 years old can take 400 to 500 mg, and adolescents 14 to 18 years old can typically take the full adult dose of 500 mg per day. This preventive use is considered off-label and should be reviewed with a pediatric healthcare provider, especially in children with kidney issues or those taking additional supplements. A buffered or chewable form may help improve tolerance, and giving it with food can reduce the risk of stomach upset.

- Early **gentle mobilization and physical therapy** is recommended. The enemy of CRPS is movement. If possible, make sure that your therapist is familiar with CRPS.

- Avoid tight-fitting braces, compression socks and boots if at all possible. After surgery, wearing a boot can help protect a child's foot or ankle, but if used for too long without movement, it may increase the risk of developing CRPS. This condition can be triggered by poor circulation, nerve irritation, or lack of movement. To help prevent CRPS, make sure the boot fits properly, encourage gentle movement of toes and nearby joints (if allowed)

- Watch out for increased abnormal pain (not normally associated with a specific surgery or injury) that is ramping up and not getting better. Also watch for skin discoloration or shine, sweating of the involved extremity, abnormal temperature of the limb or body part, extreme skin sensitivity (especially to light touch) and abnormal swelling. If ANY of these signs persist, insist that CRPS is ruled out by a knowledgeable clinician.

POTS (Postural Orthostatic Tachycardia Syndrome)

Postural Orthostatic Tachycardia Syndrome (POTS), a form of autonomic dysfunction characterized by an excessive heart rate increase upon standing, accompanied by symptoms like dizziness, fatigue, and palpitations, has been increasingly reported in pediatric populations post-COVID. Studies indicate that the viral infection may trigger dysregulation of the autonomic nervous system, leading to POTS and other dysautonomias in children and adolescents (7).

Research published in *Frontiers in Pediatrics* highlights that pediatric patients with Long COVID frequently present with symptoms overlapping with POTS, including orthostatic intolerance, exercise intolerance, and severe fatigue, which can significantly impair quality of life and school attendance (8). The pathophysiology is thought to involve immune-mediated damage, persistent inflammation, and possibly viral

Common symptoms associated with POTS in Pediatric Long COVID:

- Severe, persistent headaches

- Feeling faint or episodes of fainting

- Nausea and digestive discomfort

- Shortness of breath, even while at rest

- Crushing fatigue that does not improve with rest

- Chest pain or heart palpitations

- Weakness, blurry vision, or dizziness upon standing

Recognition of POTS in the context of Long COVID is crucial as targeted interventions—such as increased fluid and salt intake, graded exercise programs, and medications like beta-blockers or fludrocortisone—can improve symptoms and functional outcomes (9). Ongoing research is essential to better understand the mechanisms, prevalence, and optimal management strategies for pediatric Long COVID-associated POTS, underscoring the need for multidisciplinary care approaches in this vulnerable population.

FND (Functional Neurologic Disorder)

Functional Neurological Disorder (FND) has become increasingly recognized in the pediatric population, particularly in the context of post-viral syndromes such as Long COVID. Once dismissed as purely psychiatric, FND is now understood as a complex disorder of brain network dysfunction, where the nervous system has difficulty sending and receiving appropriate signals, even though no structural damage is present. Children and adolescents with FND often experience real, disabling neurological symptoms that cannot be explained by traditional medical testing. Emerging research using functional MRIs and other neuroimaging techniques has shown abnormal activity in areas of the brain responsible for movement, emotion regulation, and sensory processing—supporting FND as a neurobiological condition rather than one of malingering or attention-seeking (10).

In pediatric Long COVID cases, FND symptoms can overlap with other post-viral complications, further complicating diagnosis and treatment. A correct diagnosis and a multidisciplinary approach are essential for recovery. Most importantly, it is vital that you know that children with FND are not faking their symptoms. Their condition should be treated like any other neurological condition outside of their control. While children cannot control the symptoms of FND, they will display fewer of them when not stressed, and conversely, exhibit more symptoms when they are stressed. When your child is stressed, his or her nervous system is also under pressure. This does not mean that FND is a psychological problem that can be controlled. It cannot.

Common Symptoms of Pediatric FND in Pediatric Long COVID:

- Sudden onset of weakness or paralysis (often in limbs)

- Non-epileptic seizures (dissociative seizures)

- Abnormal movements (tremors, jerking, dystonia)

- Gait disturbances (e.g., limping, freezing, collapsing without injury)

- Sensory loss or numbness

- Speech difficulties (whispering, slurred speech, or complete loss of voice)

- Visual disturbances (blurred or tunnel vision without detectable eye pathology)

- Headaches or migraines

- Bladder or bowel disturbances without a physical cause

- Sudden, unprovoked crying or laughing (emotional dysregulation)

- Tinnitus or auditory hallucinations

- Functional tics (similar to Tourette's)

- Chest pain, dizziness, or fainting spells that mimic cardiac conditions

- Overlap with chronic fatigue or pain syndromes (e.g., fibromyalgia, AMPS, CRPS)

- Co-existing symptoms of anxiety, depression, or trauma—but not always present

Functional Neurological Disorder (FND) in pediatric patients—particularly those recovering from Long COVID—demands a shift in how we understand and approach unexplained neurological symptoms in children. No longer seen as "all in the head," FND is a real, complex condition that affects brain function and can significantly impair a child's quality of life. With early recognition, validation of the child's symptoms, and a compassionate, multidisciplinary treatment approach, many young patients can experience meaningful recovery. By continuing to educate healthcare providers and families about FND's neurobiological underpinnings, we can reduce stigma, foster healing, and ensure children receive the support and care they need.

Pediatric Acute-onset Neuropsychiatric Syndrome (PANS)

PANS is a condition where a child suddenly starts showing severe changes in behavior, mood, or physical health—often almost overnight. The changes are not caused by trauma or a known psychiatric disorder but instead by the immune system reacting to a trigger, such as an infection (including COVID-19), inflammation, or even environmental stressors. PANS can take many forms. Some children may throw things and exhibit violent and destructive behavior that is sudden and not congruent with their normal behavior.

Other children may exhibit extreme anxiety and abnormal fears and/or phobias. For instance, one of my patients, a nine-year-old little girl, developed an intense fear that someone at school would poison her food. There was no basis for this fear, and it came on suddenly after she suffered a viral infection. After early treatment in my clinic, she no longer exhibits any abnormal fear. For other kids, they may start exhibiting symptoms of obsessive-compulsive disorder. PANS is tricky as it may present in many different forms.

Think of it like this: instead of just fighting off an illness, your child's immune system accidentally affects their brain, especially areas that control emotions, behavior, and movement. This leads to very real, very distressing symptoms that can look like sudden-onset OCD, eating issues, anxiety, or even tics.

Emerging evidence indicates a connection between Pediatric Acute-onset Neuropsychiatric Syndrome (PANS) and Pediatric Long COVID. Several case reports and studies have documented instances where children developed PANS-like symptoms following SARS-CoV-2 infection. For example, a case report detailed dizygotic twin adolescents who, after asymptomatic COVID-19 infections, exhibited acute-onset obsessive-compulsive behaviors and restrictive eating patterns consistent with PANS (11).

Further research has observed that PANS symptoms triggered by COVID-19 closely resemble those initiated by other infectious agents, including obsessive-compulsive behaviors, eating disorders, and a range of emotional and behavioral symptoms (12).

Additionally, surveys and clinical observations have reported a notable number of children presenting with PANS-like symptoms following COVID-19 infection, highlighting the need for increased awareness and research into this overlap.

Common symptoms of PANS in Pediatric Long COVID:

- Sudden onset of obsessive-compulsive behaviors (OCD-like behaviors such as frequent hand-washing, checking, counting, etc.)

- Severe eating restrictions (like refusing food or fear of choking)

- Tics or other involuntary movements or sounds

- Extreme anxiety or panic attacks

- Mood swings, irritability, or aggression

- Depression or sudden sadness

- Sudden regression in learning or school performance

- Sleep disturbances (difficulty falling or staying asleep, nightmares)

- Bedwetting or frequent urination

- Sensory sensitivities (e.g., clothing feels unbearable, sounds are too loud)

- Hallucinations or delusional thinking (in more severe cases)

In my opinion, PANS is one of the most underdiagnosed and misunderstood pediatric conditions. However, if your child is suffering from PANS, please know you're not alone—and it's not your fault. PANS can be overwhelming and confusing, especially when symptoms appear suddenly and dramatically. What matters most is that you trust your instincts, seek support from knowledgeable providers, and remember that recovery is possible with the right care. Your child is still in there.

Gastrointestinal Disorders in Pediatric Long COVID:

Children recovering from COVID-19 have shown a higher risk of developing new GI tract symptoms and disorders during the post-acute phase. Gastrointestinal (GI) dysfunction is a common and often debilitating feature of pediatric Long COVID, with symptoms ranging from nausea, vomiting, abdominal pain, constipation, and diarrhea to more severe complications such as gastroparesis.

Gastroparesis, a condition where the stomach empties too slowly, has been increasingly observed in children following SARS-CoV-2 infection. This can result in persistent nausea, early satiety, bloating, and significant weight loss. In some severe cases, children may require feeding support, including nasogastric (NG) or percutaneous endoscopic gastrostomy (PEG) tubes, to maintain adequate nutrition and hydration.

One study published in *Nature Reviews Gastroenterology & Hepatology* described how SARS-CoV-2 may persist in the gut and trigger immune activation, contributing to these chronic GI symptoms (13). Similarly, research in *Frontiers in Pediatrics* documented long-term GI symptoms in pediatric Long COVID patients, noting disruptions in gut microbiota and inflammation as key factors (14). These issues not only affect physical health but also contribute to fatigue, anxiety, and school absences due to the gut-brain axis's role in systemic symptom expression. Early recognition and multidisciplinary management—including gastroenterology, nutrition, and behavioral support—are crucial for improving outcomes in these children.

Although gastrointestinal (GI) symptoms in pediatric Long COVID may seem like a purely digestive problem, emerging research shows they are often neurologically driven. The autonomic nervous system—which regulates involuntary functions like digestion—can be disrupted by SARS-CoV-2 infection, leading to dysautonomia. This dysfunction can impair gut motility, contributing to conditions like gastroparesis, where the stomach empties too slowly, causing nausea, vomiting, early satiety, and weight loss. (15)

Vagal nerve involvement has also been suggested, given its role in regulating GI function and inflammation (16). Another study specifically identified autonomic dysfunction and GI dysmotility—including gastroparesis—as common features in Long COVID patients, noting parallels with post-viral syndromes like POTS (17). These neurological disruptions may explain why some children with persistent GI symptoms require enteral nutrition despite no structural abnormalities. Recognizing GI symptoms as part of a neuroimmune and autonomic condition is essential for accurate diagnosis, compassionate care, and appropriate multidisciplinary treatment.

Here are common and serious gastrointestinal (GI) symptoms seen in pediatric Long COVID, including those related to gastroparesis:

- Nausea, especially after eating
- Vomiting (frequent or unpredictable)
- Abdominal pain or cramping
- Bloating and visible abdominal distension
- Loss of appetite
- Early satiety (feeling full after eating very little)
- Constipation or diarrhea
- Reflux or heartburn
- Food intolerance or aversion
- Weight loss or poor weight gain
- Difficulty swallowing (dysphagia)
- Malnutrition despite eating

- Dehydration from poor fluid intake or vomiting

- Severe fatigue linked to poor nutrient absorption

- Need for enteral nutrition (e.g., NG or PEG tube) due to inability to meet nutritional needs orally

- Gastroparesis (delayed stomach emptying confirmed by testing)

- Hospitalizations due to feeding complications, electrolyte imbalances, or failure to thrive

Understanding that GI issues in pediatric Long COVID are often rooted in neurologic dysfunction can be a turning point for both parents and clinicians. It shifts the narrative from one of confusion or dismissal to one of clarity and compassion. These children are not simply dealing with stomachaches—they're experiencing a breakdown in how their nervous system communicates with their gut. Recognizing this helps guide more appropriate treatments, including the use of pro-motility agents, nutritional support, and autonomic regulation strategies. Most importantly, it reinforces that these symptoms are real, biological, and deserving of care. With continued research and multidisciplinary support, there is hope for healing and recovery.

Ehlers-Danlos Syndrome (EDS)

EDS is a group of connective tissue disorders caused by defects in collagen that lead to a variety of symptoms, including joint hypermobility, skin fragility, chronic pain, and autonomic nervous system dysfunction. *Importantly, not all patients with EDS are hypermobile.* Hypermobility syndromes and EDS are related but distinct, and while many patients with EDS show hypermobility, it is not universal (18). This distinction is important when considering the overlap with Pediatric Long COVID. Doctors often mistakenly believe that all EDS patients suffer from hypermobility based on old classifications and mistakenly rule it out. It is my clinical experience that EDS is shockingly underdiagnosed.

There are 13 recognized types of EDS. Hypermobile EDS (hEDS)is the most common type of EDS. Unfortunately, no genetic marker has been identified for hEDS yet, although it is all but certain that hEDS is a genetic condition in my opinion. This makes it difficult to rule in or out hEDS. Here are some of the most common signs, symptoms and secondary conditions associated with hEDS:

Common Symptoms of Hypermobile Ehlers-Danlos Syndrome (hEDS):

- Joint instability (frequent dislocations or subluxations)
- Chronic musculoskeletal pain (affecting both bones and muscles)
- Joint pain and clicking sounds
- Constant fatigue or tiredness
- Soft, elastic skin that bruises easily
- Abnormal or slow-healing scars
- Digestive issues, such as:
  - Constipation
  - Heartburn
  - Gastroparesis (delayed stomach emptying)
- Chronic bladder infections and pain (e.g., Interstitial Cystitis)

- Autonomic nervous system dysfunctions, including:
  - Increased heart rate upon standing
  - Dizziness or lightheadedness (especially with Postural Orthostatic Tachycardia Syndrome - POTS)
- Stress incontinence (loss of bladder control)
- Internal organ issues, such as:
  - Organ prolapse
  - Mitral valve prolapse
  - Pelvic organ prolapse (especially post-pregnancy)
- Osteoporosis (reduced bone density)
- Early-onset osteoarthritis
- Joint hypermobility (excessive flexibility in large joints like knees and elbows, and small joints like fingers and toes), often painful.
- Widespread, intense pain
- Coexisting conditions (co-morbidities), such as:
  - POTS (Postural Orthostatic Tachycardia Syndrome)
  - CRPS (Complex Regional Pain Syndrome)
- Chronic anxiety
- Coinfections (often viral or bacterial, commonly underdiagnosed or missed).

It is very important to note that hypermobility *is no longer the sole or absolute criterion for diagnosing EDS.* The current 2017 international classification of EDS places emphasis on a combination of factors for diagnosing hEDS, which includes (19):

- Generalized joint hypermobility (measured by standardized scoring like the Beighton scale),

- Additional systemic manifestations of connective tissue disorder,

- Absence of other diagnoses that can better explain the symptoms,

- Family history and exclusion of other genetic causes.

Research suggests COVID-19 may trigger or worsen autonomic nervous system dysregulation, a common feature in EDS and hypermobility disorders (20).

The connection between EDS, hypermobility, and Pediatric Long COVID likely stems from immune activation, persistent inflammation, and nervous system instability caused by the viral infection, which may exacerbate underlying connective tissue vulnerabilities and autonomic dysfunction (21;22). Even patients with non-hypermobile forms of EDS may be at increased risk for prolonged or severe Long COVID symptoms due to pre-existing tissue fragility and dysautonomia (23). This overlap complicates diagnosis and treatment but highlights the need for multidisciplinary, individualized care focusing on autonomic symptom management, physical therapy, and supportive treatments.

Ongoing research aims to clarify how different EDS subtypes influence Long COVID outcomes in children and to develop targeted management strategies. Clinicians should recognize that the absence of hypermobility does not exclude EDS or connective tissue-related risks in Long COVID, emphasizing thorough assessment and personalized treatment plans.

Myalgic Encephalomyelitis/Chronic Fatigue Syndrome (ME/CFS)

ME/CFS is a complex, debilitating neuroimmune condition characterized by profound fatigue, post-exertional malaise (PEM), and cognitive and autonomic dysfunction. ME/CFS has long affected both adults and children, but following the COVID-19 pandemic, a sharp increase in ME/CFS-like symptoms has been observed in children recovering from SARS-CoV-2 infection.

ME/CFS is a serious, long-term illness that can happen after an infection like COVID-19. It's not just being tired—it's a medical condition where the body's energy systems don't work the way they should. Kids and teens with ME/CFS often feel completely worn out, even after rest. Simple things like walking to the bathroom, sitting through a class, or trying to do homework can feel overwhelming or impossible.

One of the most frustrating parts of ME/CFS is something called **post-exertional malaise (PEM)**—when doing even a small amount of physical or mental activity causes a major crash in symptoms, sometimes lasting days. These children often struggle with brain fog, body pain, sleep problems, and dizziness. On the outside, they may look "fine," but on the inside, their body is constantly struggling to keep up.

ME/CFS is not laziness, weakness, or something they can just push through. It's a medical condition involving the immune system, the nervous system, and how the body creates and uses energy. It's real—and your child is not imagining it.

Studies now confirm that Long COVID can trigger ME/CFS in both adults and pediatric populations. One study found that adolescents recovering from COVID-19 displayed persistent fatigue, cognitive dysfunction, and PEM months after infection—criteria strongly aligning with ME/CFS diagnostic guidelines (24). Another large-scale study from the UK's Office for National Statistics identified ME/CFS as a leading post-viral complication in youth with Long COVID symptoms persisting beyond 12 weeks (25).

The Institute of Medicine (IOM, now National Academy of Medicine) defined ME/CFS in 2015 as a condition with specific hallmark symptoms, which closely mirror those found in pediatric Long COVID. Recent work by Proal & VanElzakker also proposes a shared mechanism: persistent immune dysregulation, neuroinflammation, and autonomic dysfunction (26).

Common Symptoms of ME/CFS in Pediatric Long COVID:

- Severe fatigue not improved by rest
- Post-exertional malaise (PEM): worsening of symptoms after physical or mental effort
- Cognitive difficulties ("brain fog")
- Headaches and migraines
- Sleep disturbances (unrefreshing sleep, insomnia)
- Dizziness or lightheadedness (especially when standing)
- Sensitivity to light, sound, or touch
- Muscle and joint pain
- Nausea or digestive symptoms
- Difficulty concentrating in school or returning to normal activities
- Autonomic dysfunction (including POTS)

- Temperature dysregulation (feeling too hot or too cold)

- Emotional lability or mood changes (often due to
  neurological fatigue)

For families walking through the storm of pediatric Long COVID, hearing your child describe relentless exhaustion, brain fog, or pain with no clear explanation can be frightening and frustrating. ME/CFS is very real—it's not "just in their head" or something they can push through with more effort. Understanding that this is a neuroimmune condition with clear biological underpinnings helps bring compassion and legitimacy to your child's experience. There is hope in the growing body of research, and with validation, pacing strategies, supportive care, and the right therapies, many children find stability and even recovery. You are not alone— and neither is your child.

While the journey through pediatric Long COVID can be overwhelming and filled with uncertainty, it is important to remember that you are not alone, and neither is your child. The physical, emotional, and neurological effects of this condition are very real, but so is the growing awareness, research, and medical support surrounding it. More clinicians are learning how to recognize and treat these symptoms, and more families are speaking out and finding community in shared experience. Recovery may not follow a straight line, but with patience, the right care, and a team that listens and believes you, healing is possible.

Just as importantly, parents need to be aware of the other conditions that may develop alongside or after Long COVID, such as POTS, ME/CFS, CRPS, AMPS, FND, and more. These aren't rare in this context—and knowing what to look for can save families months or even years of frustration, misdiagnosis, or being dismissed by doctors who simply don't yet understand. When you know what's possible, you can advocate early, seek the right specialists, and help your child get the care they deserve.

Chapter 4:
When The World Doesn't See: The Emotional Impact Of Parenting A Child With An Invisible Illness

"To be a mother of a sick child is to walk through fire, every day, and pretend you're not burning."

Anonymous

"What hurts the most is not being seen or heard when you are hurting."

Unknown

A Silent Grief

No one ever dreams of sitting in a hospital waiting room, researching symptoms late into the night, or watching their child fade from the inside out while the world shrugs. But here you are. Not by choice. Not because you did something wrong. But because something unthinkable happened, and your child got sick.

And now, you are in the space between worlds. In one world, there are friends, family, doctors—even teachers—who often don't see what you see. They question it. Minimize it. Ignore it. In the other world, your child is suffering—chronically, silently, and often invisibly. Their joy, energy, and abilities have changed. Sometimes their very personality has shifted. And you, as their parent, live in both worlds at once—witnessing and advocating, believing and grieving.

This chapter is for you.

The Emotional Toll on Parents and Caregivers

When your child is living with an invisible illness like Pediatric Long COVID, the emotional impact on you as a parent or caregiver can be just as overwhelming and painful as the illness itself. Unlike visible injuries or conditions, invisible diseases carry the added burden of misunderstanding—from the outside world and sometimes even from those closest to you. The stress, exhaustion, and heartbreak you experience can feel endless and isolating.

You may find yourself grappling with a mix of emotions that shift day to day, or even hour to hour, including:

- **Powerlessness:** Watching your child struggle with symptoms that you cannot fix or fully understand is a unique and profound helplessness. You want to protect them, to make it better, but often all you can do is bear witness to their pain and hope for answers.

- **Anger:** Frustration with the medical system is common. You may feel anger toward doctors who dismiss symptoms, insurance companies that deny coverage, or even well-meaning friends and family who suggest your child's suffering is "all in their head." This anger is valid and often arises from feeling unheard and unsupported.

- **Isolation:** Many parents report feeling deeply alone on this journey. Friends may drift away because they don't understand or because social gatherings become too difficult. Even family members might minimize the illness or imply that you're overreacting. This isolation compounds the emotional burden.

- **Guilt:** You may wrestle with guilt for not recognizing symptoms sooner, for not being able to do more, or for struggling to balance caregiving with other aspects of your life. These feelings are natural, but do not reflect your true dedication or love.

- **Exhaustion:** The physical, emotional, and spiritual toll of caregiving can drain every ounce of energy. Sleepless nights, constant vigilance, and the mental strain of advocating for your child take a heavy toll on your well-being.

- **Grief:** There is a profound grief—not only for the health your child once had, but also for the life you imagined for them and the family you envisioned. It's a mourning for lost normalcy and the dreams deferred by chronic illness.

As one mother shared, *"I felt so alone for the longest time. It was like no one believed us—like we were making it all up. That hurt worse than the illness sometimes."* Your feelings are completely normal and valid. You are carrying a weight that few outside your experience can truly understand.

Studies have shown that caregivers of children with chronic invisible illnesses experience significantly higher rates of anxiety, depression, and caregiver burnout compared to the general population (1). The uncertainty of the illness's course, combined with societal misunderstanding and skepticism, only intensifies the emotional strain (2). Recognizing these feelings is the first step toward healing and finding ways to support both you and your child through this difficult journey.

Navigating the Emotional Journey: Practical Advice for Parents and Caregivers

While the path you're on is undeniably challenging, there are strategies that can help you protect your emotional well-being and advocate effectively for your child:

- **Build a Support Network:** Seek out other parents and caregivers who understand what you're going through. Online support groups, local chronic illness communities, and organizations dedicated to Pediatric Long COVID can provide invaluable empathy and advice.

- **Prioritize Self-Care:** Remember that caring for yourself is essential—not selfish. Try to carve out moments for rest, hobbies, or simple pleasures, even if brief. Small acts of self-kindness recharge your capacity to care for your child.

- **Practice Mindfulness and Stress Reduction:** Techniques like deep breathing, meditation, or gentle yoga can help reduce anxiety and improve emotional resilience. Apps and online resources can guide you if you're new to these practices.

- **Educate Yourself and Others:** Learning as much as you can about Pediatric Long COVID empowers you to be your child's best advocate. Sharing accurate information with family and friends can sometimes reduce misunderstandings.

- **Set Boundaries:** It's okay to limit contact with people who are unsupportive or dismissive. Protect your family's emotional space to preserve your energy.

- **Communicate Openly with Your Child:** Age-appropriate honesty about their illness and feelings fosters trust and helps your child feel less alone. Validate their experiences and encourage them to express their emotions.

- **Seek Professional Help:** Don't hesitate to reach out to mental health professionals experienced with chronic illness families. Counseling or therapy can provide coping tools and a safe space to process grief and frustration.

- **Celebrate Small Victories:** Acknowledge every positive step, no matter how small. Progress in symptom management, a good day, or a moment of joy are important milestones.

Remember, you are not alone in this journey. Your love and dedication are powerful forces, and by taking care of yourself, you strengthen your ability to support your child through the uncertainties of Pediatric Long COVID.

Helping Your Child Face a Disbelieving World

One of the most heartbreaking challenges of parenting a child with an invisible illness like Pediatric Long COVID is witnessing how disbelief from others can deeply wound your child. When friends, family members, teachers, or even healthcare providers question the reality of their symptoms, it can erode your child's self-esteem, damage their sense of safety, and sometimes even diminish their hope and motivation to keep fighting.

Why This Matters:

Invisible illnesses are often misunderstood because they lack obvious physical signs. This makes your child's pain and struggle easy to dismiss or minimize by those who have never experienced it. Unfortunately, these doubts can leave your child feeling isolated and invisible on top of their physical suffering.

Ways You Can Help Your Child Navigate This:

1. Believe Them Fiercely

Your unwavering belief is the most vital foundation your child needs. They must know you see and hear their experience clearly and without judgment. Tell them often, in words and actions:

- *"I believe you."*

- *"You are not making this up."*

- *"I see how hard this is for you."*

Hearing this reassurance repeatedly helps your child trust themselves and counters the damaging messages from others.

2. Model Self-Advocacy

Children learn by watching you. When you stand up for their needs—whether with doctors, teachers, or relatives—your child gains a powerful lesson in how to assert themselves respectfully but firmly. This might mean:

- Asking doctors thorough questions

- Requesting accommodations at school

- Correcting misinformation from relatives or friends

By calmly modeling these behaviors, you teach your child to advocate for their health and well-being in a world that often doesn't understand invisible illness.

3. Validate Their Emotional Experience

Invisible illness impacts more than just the body. Your child may feel overwhelmed by fear, confusion, sadness, or anger. Validating these feelings helps your child process them instead of hiding or suppressing them. Try saying:

- *"It makes sense that you feel scared."*

- *"It's okay to be mad about what you're going through."*

- *"I'm here with you, no matter how you feel."*

This emotional validation is key to building resilience and trust.

4. Protect Their Peace

Not everyone in your child's life will be supportive or understanding. People who gaslight (deny your child's experience), undermine, or minimize their symptoms can do real harm. It's important to:

- Set boundaries around contact with these individuals

- Limit exposure to negative or dismissive conversations

- Shield your child's emotional space as much as possible, even if the person is family

This protection helps preserve your child's mental health and sense of security.

5. Help Them Find Their People

Finding others who "get it" can transform your child's experience. Look for:

- Local or online support groups for children with Long COVID or chronic illness

- Social media communities where kids share their stories and encouragement

- Activities or groups where your child can connect with peers facing similar challenges

Belonging to a community reduces feelings of isolation and builds hope.

Resources for Parents and Children

- **Solve ME/CFS Initiative (SMCI):** Offers resources and support for families dealing with chronic fatigue syndrome and similar illnesses, including pediatric patients. solvecfs.org

- **Long COVID Kids:** A UK-based charity providing educational resources, advocacy, and support groups specifically for children and families dealing with Long COVID. longcovidkids.org

- **The Mighty:** An online community with groups for children and teens with chronic illness, including Long COVID, where your child can connect and share stories. themighty.com

- **Chronic Illness Peer Support Groups:** Local hospitals or pediatric clinics may offer support groups for children with chronic illness and their families—ask your provider for referrals.

- **School Advocacy Organizations:** Groups like the National Center for Learning Disabilities (ncld.org) provide tools and guidance on securing accommodations and rights for children with invisible illnesses in educational settings.

By fiercely believing in your child, teaching them to stand up for themselves, validating their feelings, protecting their emotional safety, and helping them connect with understanding peers and support networks, you can help your child face the outside world with courage and hope—even when it feels like no one else understands.

Speaking to Siblings and Extended Family

When a child has an invisible illness like Pediatric Long COVID, it doesn't just affect that child—it ripples throughout the entire family. Siblings and extended family members often struggle to understand what's happening. Their feelings range widely—from confusion and jealousy to worry and even guilt. As a parent or caregiver, you play a crucial role in helping your family navigate these complex emotions with empathy and clear communication.

Educate with Compassion

Not everyone will immediately grasp the reality of Long COVID, especially in children, where symptoms are invisible and fluctuating. But many family members genuinely want to understand if given the chance. Sharing trustworthy resources can bridge this gap:

- Articles and books written specifically for families about pediatric Long COVID can demystify the illness and dispel myths.

- Documentaries or videos that show real stories of children living with chronic illness make the invisible visible and build empathy.

- Encourage extended family to ask questions and express their concerns without judgment, and gently correct misinformation.

Remember, education is most effective when it comes from a place of patience and understanding, not blame or frustration.

Set Clear Boundaries

It's essential to protect your child—and your family—from disbelief or dismissiveness that can be hurtful and damaging. Setting firm boundaries is an act of love and self-care.
You might say:

- *"We don't tolerate people doubting our child's illness."*

- *"If you can't be supportive, please respect our need for space."*

- Enforce these boundaries consistently, even with close relatives. This sends a clear message that your child's experience is valid and non-negotiable.

Healthy boundaries prevent toxic dynamics and preserve your child's emotional safety.

Give Siblings Space to Feel

Siblings often experience a whirlwind of emotions that can be confusing and difficult to express. They may:

- Feel neglected as much attention and resources go toward the sick child.

- Be worried about their sibling's health but unsure how to help.

- Experience guilt for being healthy or frustration over changes in family routines.

Including siblings as much as possible helps them feel seen and valued. This can be as simple as:

- Setting aside time just for them, even if brief.

- Talking openly and honestly about what's happening, using age-appropriate language.

- Encouraging them to share their feelings without fear of judgment.

- Empowering them to participate in caregiving in small ways which can foster connection and purpose.

By acknowledging siblings' feelings, you build family resilience and prevent resentment or isolation. Navigating invisible illness in the family requires both education and emotional sensitivity. By compassionately informing siblings and extended family, setting firm boundaries to protect your child, and creating space for siblings' feelings, you foster a supportive family environment where everyone's experience is honored. This holistic approach not only strengthens your child with Long COVID but also helps your entire family weather the challenges together.

The Heartache of Being the Parent of a Child with Invisible, Daily Struggles

I want to speak directly to one of the most deeply affected groups in Pediatric Long COVID—the parents and caregivers. It doesn't matter if your child is a toddler or a teenager; the pain of watching them suffer day after day is a unique kind of heartache. As a parent myself, I believe there is little more devastating than witnessing your child struggle with an illness that the world often cannot see or understand.

In my conversations with the brave parents of children with Long COVID, I hear stories that both break my heart and fill me with admiration. Stories of missed birthdays, canceled school events, and lost friendships. Stories of children too fatigued to play outside, too foggy to focus in class, and too overwhelmed to engage in the life they once loved. These parents watch other families move forward while their child remains stuck in a fog of symptoms and uncertainty. At night, they worry not only about today, but about their child's future.

Questions haunt you that other parents may never have to ask:

- Will my child ever regain their energy and joy?
- Will they find friends who understand?
- Will they have careers, relationships, and independence?
- Who will care for them when I am no longer able to?

Your experience is often misunderstood except by others walking this same painful path. Your grief can feel isolating, a quiet storm no one else fully sees.

When you share your child's medical history with doctors or therapists, it's often with a careful, practiced calm—because you've done this countless times before. You don't want pity. You don't want sympathy. You have learned to build a protective wall around your heart because if it cracks, your sorrow might overwhelm you. You cannot afford to drown in grief—not when your child needs your strength and presence every day.

You fight fiercely for your child's care and well-being. You spend your energy, your resources, and your hope because this is your child, and you were chosen to protect them.

I see you. I admire you. I know you did not choose this path, but you are walking it with courage and grace. You are the steadfast pillar your child leans on, the unwavering force that holds them up. Your love is the most powerful medicine they have.

As a parent, I cannot imagine a more difficult reality than standing helplessly beside your child as they endure persistent, invisible symptoms. Please know my heart goes out to you. This is one of life's hardest challenges.

You want only what's best for your child—safety, happiness, and health. Yet sometimes, life delivers battles no one prepares us for. Pediatric Long COVID is one of those battles.

In this struggle, your role is clear but demanding: become your child's strongest advocate and greatest source of strength. This will require resilience beyond what you thought possible.

It is natural to scream "Why?!" in moments of despair. But illness and fatigue cannot be wished away by sheer will or love alone. Instead, become informed, stay steady, and be the unshakable support your child needs in their hardest moments.

I want to share a personal story of strength from my own family: When my niece Mia was born with a heart condition, she underwent open-heart surgery at five weeks old. My sister, a physician herself, faced this terrifying ordeal largely on her own. Through this, I learned what true strength looks like. She never let her fear show but channeled every ounce of it into fighting for Mia's life. She learned the complex medical machinery and became a fierce advocate, turning obstacles into opportunities for growth. Today, Mia is a spirited little warrior, confident and joyful—a testament to the power of a parent's love and determination.

Your child will have moments of sadness and anger, and it's okay for them to lean on you sometimes. But your role is to hold their pain without being consumed by it. They need a safe harbor in a world made uncertain by their illness. They need you to be strong when they feel weak.

Find sources of support and energy for yourself—friends, counselors, or communities—so you can recharge and show up fully for your child.

Children with chronic, invisible illnesses often carry deep guilt for the impact their condition has on the family. It's crucial to remind them that they are not defined by their symptoms. Their presence is a gift, a light that enriches your life and your family's, no matter the challenges.

Counseling can be a vital tool—not only for your child but for your family's relationships, including siblings who may feel overlooked or confused.

Your family will face obstacles that many others cannot imagine. But these obstacles can also be a source of resilience, connection, and unexpected strength. I believe in your ability to walk this path with courage.

Know this: Your child chose you. Their soul recognized a strength within you and entrusted you with this sacred role. It is an incredible privilege and responsibility. As the poet Kahlil Gibran said, *"Your children are not your children. They are the sons and daughters of Life's longing for itself. They come through you but not from you. And though they are with you, yet they belong not to you."*

Your child's journey is intertwined with yours in a story of love, struggle, and enduring hope.

Taking Care of Yourself Without Guilt

As a parent or caregiver of a child with an invisible illness like Pediatric Long COVID, it's easy to lose yourself in the whirlwind of appointments, treatments, and endless emotional labor. But your well-being is not a luxury — it's essential. You matter, too. Caring for yourself isn't selfish; it's necessary so that you can keep showing up for your child and your family.

You don't have to carry this burden alone. It is crucial that you find support. Find someone—or some space—where you can simply be heard and supported, without pressure to "fix" everything. This could be:

- A **therapist or counselor** who understands chronic illness and caregiving fatigue.

- A **close friend** who listens without judgment and lets you vent your raw feelings.

- A **parent support group**, especially one focused on invisible or chronic illnesses, where others truly understand what you're going through. Allowing yourself to be held emotionally is not a sign of weakness—it's an act of strength and self-preservation.

Make Room for Joy

Even during the darkest, most overwhelming days, small moments of joy can be lifelines. These moments don't have to be grand or time-consuming—sometimes just five minutes is enough to reset your spirit. Consider:

- Savoring a cup of coffee or tea outside in the fresh air.

- Taking a short, quiet walk alone where you can breathe deeply.

- Watching a funny show or reading a book that transports you somewhere lighter.

- Listening to music that lifts your mood or calms your nerves.

These "pockets of light" are what will sustain you through the long journey. They remind you that life still holds beauty and hope, even when it's hard to see.

This situation is unlike anything you or anyone else anticipated. There is no perfect way to parent a child with a complex, invisible illness. You are doing your absolute best, navigating uncertainty and challenges every day—and that is enough. It is time to let go of the plans you had and to stop grieving. Release the impossible expectations of being "supermom," "superdad," or "supercaregiver." Your love and effort matter far more than any checklist or external judgment.

The Light That Comes Through the Cracks

Your child's illness may be a heavy part of your story now, but it is not all they are — and it is not all you are. This difficult path you walk together is shaping something powerful within both of you.

Through your steadfast belief in your child's truth, you are teaching them invaluable lessons:

- **Resilience**—how to keep going even when the world doubts or misunderstands.

- **Courage**—to speak their truth loudly and clearly, no matter the resistance.

- **Love**—the kind that holds steady in the face of pain and uncertainty.

Your child will learn what real love looks like—not from those who accepted their illness easily, but from a parent who believed against all odds, who stood as their fiercest advocate and safe harbor. Yes, this journey is unfair. It is exhausting and heartbreaking. But you are not alone. And your child is not alone.

Together, you are weaving a story that is both painful and profoundly powerful. One that shines a light for others who will walk this path after you. You are part of a community bound by courage, hope, and unshakable love.

Chapter 5:
The Neurologic Link

"All body systems would be immobilized without the nervous system. It controls and regulates every bodily activity down to the workings of the tiniest cell."

World Book Encyclopedia of Medicine

"Your immune cells are like a circulating nervous system. Your nervous system, in fact, is a circulating nervous system. It thinks. It's conscious."

Deepak Chopra

The Autonomic Nervous System and Pediatric Long COVID

The autonomic nervous system (ANS) is like your child's body's autopilot—it keeps everything running smoothly without them even thinking about it. It controls their heart rate, digestion, blood pressure, breathing, and even how they respond to stress. But when Long COVID affects the ANS, this vital system can get thrown off balance, leading to a wide range of frustrating and sometimes scary symptoms.

Our healthcare system often focuses on managing symptoms rather than finding the root cause of a problem. This means kids with Long COVID are often given medications to mask pain, calm dizziness, or improve sleep—but these don't fix the underlying issue. While symptom relief is important, true healing happens when we help the body regain balance and restore function, not just cover up discomfort.

Think of the autonomic nervous system like a highly advanced computer program running in the background of your child's body. It keeps every system functioning properly without them having to think about it. Now imagine a virus crashing that program. Systems start malfunctioning, signals get crossed, and basic functions become unpredictable. This is what happens when Long COVID disrupts the ANS. It's also why children with Long COVID often experience a mix of symptoms—racing hearts, dizziness, stomach issues, temperature regulation problems, and extreme fatigue. Their nervous system is struggling to find balance.

One of the biggest concerns is that this nervous system dysfunction can also impact the immune system, making it harder for the body to fight off infections and heal properly. This connection between the nervous system and the immune system is crucial to understanding how Long COVID affects children.

The Nervous System and the Immune System: A Critical Connection

At first, scientists thought the immune system and the brain only communicated indirectly through chemical signals in the bloodstream. Over time, research has shown that the brain and immune system are directly linked, working together in ways that are still being discovered. When one is out of balance, the other is affected.

Cytokines—tiny proteins that help the immune system communicate—play a key role in this connection. They help regulate inflammation, signal when to fight infections, and assist in healing. However, when Long COVID disrupts the nervous system, cytokine levels can become abnormal, leading to ongoing inflammation, immune exhaustion, and problems in multiple body systems.

The immune system acts like a team of security guards, constantly patrolling the body for threats and calling for reinforcements when needed. It learns from past infections and builds stronger defenses over time. This network includes the thymus, bone marrow, spleen, lymph nodes, tonsils, and even the skin. Given how closely these organs work together, it makes sense that the immune system and nervous system must communicate effectively for overall health.

When this communication breaks down, it can contribute to a range of health issues—including Long COVID. Scientists now know that immune cells and the nervous system interact in ways that affect everything from inflammation to mental health. If these pathways are disrupted, children can experience ongoing immune system problems, mood changes, and increased susceptibility to infections.

Immune Exhaustion: A Key Factor in Pediatric Long COVID?

The immune system is designed to ramp up when fighting an infection and then return to normal. However, in some Long COVID cases, the immune system gets stuck in an overactive state, leading to exhaustion. Research shows that some children with Long COVID have dramatically low levels of key cytokines, including IFNγ and IL-8, as well as reductions in IL-2, IL-4, IL-6, IL-13, and IL-17 (1). This suggests their immune system is running on empty.

IL-8, for example, plays a crucial role in calling white blood cells to damaged areas to assist with healing. If IL-8 levels are depleted, tissues—like those in the lungs—may struggle to recover properly after an initial COVID infection. This could explain lingering symptoms like persistent cough, shortness of breath, fatigue, and post-exertional malaise (a worsening of symptoms after physical or mental activity).

Understanding immune exhaustion in children with Long COVID is a significant step toward better treatment. If the immune system is depleted, children may not just be dealing with lingering symptoms but with a deeper, unresolved immune imbalance that needs targeted support to recover.

The Path Forward

Long COVID is still being studied, and new discoveries are emerging. What we do know is that the nervous system and immune system are deeply connected, and their dysfunction plays a major role in lingering symptoms. The key to helping children recover lies in addressing this imbalance—not just managing symptoms but restoring the body's ability to heal itself.

As parents, caregivers, and advocates, understanding these mechanisms can empower you to seek better care for your child. While symptom relief is important, true healing means finding and addressing the root causes. The more we learn, the more we can push for research, treatments, and medical approaches that prioritize full recovery—not just temporary fixes.

Your child's body is resilient. With the right approach, balance can be restored, and healing can begin.

The Vagus Nerve and Pediatric Long COVID

(For more information about healing the vagus nerve, please read "Accessing the Healing Power of the Vagus Nerve" by Stanley Rosenberg. I found it to be one of the most helpful and brilliant books on this topic available today.)

The vagus nerve is one of the most important nerves in your child's body, acting as a communication superhighway between the brain, immune system, heart, lungs, and digestive system. It plays a key role in helping the body regulate inflammation, digestion, heart rate, and even emotional responses. If the vagus nerve isn't working properly, a child can experience issues with breathing, swallowing, digestion, heart function, and overall immune health. When Long COVID affects the vagus nerve, it can disrupt multiple body systems at once, leading to a wide range of symptoms.

The Vagus Nerve: The Body's Master Communicator

The vagus nerve is constantly sending information back and forth between the brain and body. About 80% of the signals travel *upward* from the body to the brain (afferent signals), while the remaining 20% travel downward from the brain to the body (afferent signals). This means that the brain relies heavily on the vagus nerve to understand what's happening inside the body and respond appropriately.

In simpler terms, the vagus nerve is like the messenger between the brain and the rest of the body. When this messenger is disrupted—such as by a viral infection—the brain can receive faulty information about what's going on inside the body, leading to problems like chronic inflammation, digestive issues, brain fog, and nervous system dysregulation.

The Vagus Nerve and Immune Function

Many parents tell me they've tried countless treatments, supplements, and therapies to help their child recover from Long COVID, but nothing seems to work. The reason? They may be trying to "clean the pond" without fixing the broken fountain.

Think of the immune system as a pond, and the vagus nerve as the fountain that keeps the water moving. If the fountain stops working, the water in the pond becomes stagnant, allowing bacteria, viruses, and toxins to build up. You can clean the pond over and over again, but unless you fix the fountain, the water will become dirty again in no time. Healing the vagus nerve is key to restoring immune balance.

Dr. Kevin Tracey and his team at Northwell Health's Feinstein Institutes discovered that the vagus nerve plays a critical role in controlling inflammation. This nerve is a key part of the inflammatory reflex system, which helps the immune system fight infections without overreacting and damaging healthy cells.

When an infection enters the body, immune cells send signals through the vagus nerve to alert the brain. The brain then allocates resources to combat the infection, and once the threat is eliminated, the vagus nerve instructs the immune system to return to a balanced state.

But what happens if the vagus nerve isn't working properly? Inflammation stays active for too long. This can cause ongoing symptoms like fatigue, brain fog, pain, and digestive problems—all common in children with Long COVID.

The Vagus Nerve and Viral Invasion

Some viruses—including COVID-19—have the ability to hijack the vagus nerve and use it as a pathway into the brain. This is especially concerning because the vagus nerve is deeply connected to the lungs, heart, and digestive system—all areas where COVID-19 is known to cause damage.

COVID-19 can bind to acetylcholine (ACh) receptors, which are crucial for immune function, nerve communication, and blood flow regulation. ACh acts like a chemical messenger, sending signals between the brain and body. If a virus interferes with these signals, the nervous system can become dysregulated, leading to symptoms like:

- Breathing difficulties
- Heart rate irregularities
- Severe fatigue
- Brain fog and memory issues
- Digestive problems
- Widespread inflammation

How COVID-19 Gets Into the Brain

The debate over how COVID-19 enters the brain is ongoing, but scientists agree that it can and does happen (2). Here are some of the main ways the virus can reach the brain and nervous system:

1. Through the Vagus Nerve (The "Ladder to the Brain")

COVID-19 has been found in lung tissue, blood vessels, and muscle tissue in the respiratory tract (3,4). Since the vagus nerve is directly connected to the lungs, it may serve as a pathway for the virus to travel into the brain. Once inside, the virus can cause brain inflammation, neurological dysfunction, and long-term nervous system dysregulation.

2. Through the Olfactory Nerve (The "Nose Gateway")

The olfactory nerve, which controls our sense of smell, is one of the most well-known entry points for COVID-19 into the brain (5). This nerve is located close to the hippocampus, which controls memory, learning, and emotional regulation. This could explain why so many children with Long COVID experience brain fog, mood changes, and cognitive issues.

3. Through the Gut (The "Second Brain")

The gut and brain are deeply connected through the gut-brain axis, a two-way communication system between the digestive system and the nervous system. Inside the gut, there are millions of good and bad bacteria that play a role in immune health, digestion, and even mood regulation. When the gut is out of balance, it can lead to symptoms like anxiety, depression, weight gain, food sensitivities, and autoimmune issues.

COVID-19 can disrupt the gut microbiome, leading to inflammation, immune dysfunction, and even neurological symptoms. Some studies show that even a single round of antibiotics can cause changes in gut bacteria that lead to anxiety and depression (6). This highlights the importance of restoring gut health as part of healing from Long COVID.

The Blood-Brain Barrier: The Body's "Castle Wall"

The blood-brain barrier (BBB) is like a castle wall, protecting the brain from harmful invaders. But research shows that COVID-19 can breach this barrier, allowing viruses, toxins, and inflammatory molecules to enter the brain (7).

One study found that the BBB was disrupted in 58% of COVID-19 patients with neurological symptoms (8), and this damage may last for a long time (9). When the brain is unprotected, it becomes more vulnerable to future infections, inflammation, and neurological problems.

The Path Forward

Understanding the vagus nerve's role in Long COVID gives us powerful insight into how to help children recover.

- If the vagus nerve is weak, the immune system can become overactive, leading to chronic inflammation.

- If the gut-brain connection is disrupted, it can affect mood, energy levels, and digestion.

- If the blood-brain barrier is damaged, the brain can become more vulnerable to infections and inflammation.

The good news? The vagus nerve can heal with the right interventions. By focusing on restoring nervous system function, immune balance, and gut health, we can help children with Long COVID reclaim their health and vitality.

Long COVID is complex, but every piece of knowledge brings us closer to solutions. Your child's body is resilient. With the right tools, healing is possible.

Further Consequences of Viral Invasion

Unfortunately, the damage doesn't end once COVID-19 enters the central nervous system (CNS). It can cause ongoing issues long after the initial infection. Research has shown that coronaviruses have been found in human brain samples after death (10), proving that these viruses, while primarily affecting the respiratory system, are also naturally neuroinvasive (16). Even more concerning, COVID-19 can replicate itself inside the brain and may cause a long-term infection within CNS cells.

Hypoxia: When the Brain Doesn't Get Enough Oxygen

COVID-19 affects the lungs, making it harder for the body to get enough oxygen—a condition called hypoxia. This lack of oxygen can impact the brain in serious ways, including strokes, seizures, cognitive impairment, and even permanent brain damage. Many symptoms of Long COVID may be tied to this lack of oxygen.

Hypoxia is also linked to increased inflammation (11), which is responsible for a range of conditions, including heart disease, autoimmune disorders, and chronic pain. Additionally, damage to tiny blood vessels can result in tissue damage anywhere in the body.

Severe cases of COVID-19 that required ICU hospitalization have shown significant brain damage in some patients (12), reinforcing the need to address Long COVID's impact on the brain.

Secondary Infections: When Other Illnesses Take Advantage

Once the body's defenses are weakened, other harmful invaders can take over. One example is encephalitis, a dangerous brain inflammation often caused by the herpes simplex virus. Some COVID-19 patients have also been affected by rhino-orbital mucormycosis, a rare but deadly fungal infection, particularly those with type II diabetes or those treated with steroids during COVID-19.

COVID-19 has also been linked to the reactivation of dormant viruses in the body, such as Epstein-Barr virus (EBV), which can cause prolonged fatigue and other complications (13).

Understanding the Polyvagal Theory:

Why the Nervous System Gets "Stuck"

To understand how COVID-19 affects the autonomic nervous system (ANS), we must first explore the Polyvagal Theory. Dr. Stephen Porges introduced this concept in 1994, offering a groundbreaking view of how the vagus nerve functions.

His research suggests that the ANS isn't just about two opposing states—fight-or-flight (sympathetic) versus rest-and-digest (parasympathetic). Instead, he proposed a three-part system:

1. **Dorsal Vagus Nerve:** This branch, originating in the back of the brainstem, is unmyelinated (lacking an insulating sheath), which slows down nerve signal transmission. When triggered, it can cause a shutdown response—similar to an animal "playing dead" when under attack. This state can leave a child feeling exhausted, withdrawn, and socially disconnected. When prolonged, it can lead to depression, digestive issues, and a general loss of motivation. However, when balanced with a healthy nervous system, this state can also support deep relaxation and recovery.

2. **Ventral Vagus Nerve:** Originating in the front of the brainstem, this myelinated branch allows for social connection, emotional regulation, and overall well-being. It is linked to restful sleep, healthy breathing, and proper digestion. A well-functioning ventral vagus nerve helps a child feel calm and safe.

3. **Sympathetic Chain:** This system prepares the body for danger by increasing heart rate, blood pressure, and alertness. When overactive, it can cause constant anxiety, fear, and restlessness—leading to exhaustion over time.

Why the Vagus Nerve Matters for Long COVID

For children dealing with Long COVID, one of the biggest challenges is when the autonomic nervous system—the part of the nervous system that controls things your child doesn't have to think about, like heart rate, digestion, and breathing—gets out of balance. Normally, this system helps the body respond quickly to danger by triggering the fight-or-flight response, and then it settles back down when the danger passes. But in Long COVID, the system can get "stuck" in this stress mode, leaving a child's body on high alert all the time. This constant stress can cause problems like ongoing anxiety, trouble sleeping, weaker immune defenses, and exhaustion from the adrenal glands working too hard.

Many medical treatments focus on individual symptoms—like giving medicine for anxiety or sleep problems—without addressing the bigger problem: the nervous system itself being out of sync. If the nervous system remains stuck in overdrive, these treatments might help a little, but they often don't fix the root cause. That's why children with Long COVID may continue to struggle despite various medications or therapies.

A common feature of Long COVID is something called chronic dysautonomia, where the autonomic nervous system can't properly regulate itself. This is where the vagus nerve plays a key role. The vagus nerve is like a major highway in the nervous system, connecting the brain to many important organs and helping to control the body's rest-and-digest functions. Activating the ventral part of the vagus nerve—one of its main pathways—can help "reset" this whole system and bring much-needed balance back to the body.

When the ventral vagus nerve is stimulated, it encourages other important nerves in the head and neck (like cranial nerves V, VII, and IX) to start working properly again, improving communication between the brain and body. This can lead to better regulation of heart rate, digestion, breathing, and emotional responses. For children with Long COVID, therapies that support vagus nerve function can reduce anxiety, improve sleep, strengthen immune responses, and boost energy levels, helping their bodies find calm and healing after months of chaos.

Understanding the role of the vagus nerve gives parents and caregivers a clearer picture of why symptoms happen and points to therapies that target the nervous system's balance—not just the symptoms. Supporting the vagus nerve is an important step toward helping children regain control of their bodies and feel like themselves again. It's a hopeful and powerful piece of the healing puzzle for pediatric Long COVID.

Common Nervous System Issues in Long COVID

Many Long COVID patients report dysfunctions related to cranial nerves, which can cause:

- Trigeminal neuralgia (intense facial pain) (14)

- Loss of taste or smell

- Difficulty swallowing

- Changes in voice

- Digestive problems

- Chronic anxiety and depression

How to Help the Nervous System Heal

Activating the ventral vagus nerve can improve many of these symptoms. Think of it as a see-saw—when the ventral vagus nerve is stimulated, it naturally balances the other branches of the nervous system.

In our clinic, we use specialized manual vagus nerve activation performed by trained professionals. However, there are simple ways to activate the vagus nerve at home, including:

- Gargling

- Humming or singing

- Splashing cold water on the face

Additionally, a device called the Rezzimax can be highly effective for vagus nerve stimulation. This handheld tool delivers specialized vibrations that help reset the nervous system. For more information, visit www.rezzimax.com and look for instructional videos on social media.

Channelopathy and Long COVID in Children

Our bodies rely on tiny structures called ion channels to keep cells working properly. You can think of these channels like garage doors in the walls of cells. When the doors open, important particles (called ions) move in and out. These include sodium, potassium, calcium, and chloride. Each type has a special job: sodium helps "spark" signals, potassium balances them out, calcium controls muscle and nerve activity, and chloride helps keep everything stable. Together, this flow of ions creates the electrical signals that allow nerves to send messages, muscles to contract, and organs to function smoothly.

A channelopathy happens when these garage doors don't open or close the way they should. Instead of moving smoothly, they may get stuck open, closed, or open at the wrong time. This causes mixed-up signals in the body. For example:

- **Potassium channels** help "reset" the nerve signal after it fires. If they don't work right, the signal can get louder or longer than it should—almost like turning up the volume on a speaker. This may explain why some children feel pain more intensely or for longer periods.

- **Sodium channels** act like the spark that starts a message. If they become overactive, nerves may fire too often, leading to tingling, burning, or muscle twitching.

- **Calcium channels** control how nerves talk to each other. When these are unstable, communication between brain cells may become uncoordinated, leading to problems with concentration, memory, or even mood.

- **Chloride channels** act like stabilizers, preventing nerves from firing too easily. When they are off balance, children may experience muscle stiffness, fatigue, or difficulty relaxing.

COVID-19 and its lingering effects may interfere with these ion channels in two main ways. First, the immune system's response to the virus can cause inflammation, which jams or warps the garage doors so they don't open and close properly. Second, some studies suggest the virus may directly damage the proteins that form the "motors" and "springs" of these doors. When this happens, normal rhythms, like nerve signals, heartbeats, or blood pressure regulation, become unstable.

Because ion channels are found all throughout the body, channelopathies can create a wide variety of symptoms. In pediatric Long COVID, this might look like dizziness when standing, difficulty concentrating ("brain fog"), unexplained muscle aches, or sudden fatigue. This also explains why symptoms can shift from day to day or move from one system to another. It's not just one organ that's affected, but the communication network itself.

When ion channels (those tiny "garage doors" in nerve cells) don't open and close properly, the result can be nerve over-excitability. Sodium channels may spark too often, while potassium channels that normally "quiet" the signal fail to calm it down. This imbalance makes pain pathways behave like an amplifier stuck on high volume, turning normal sensations or small signals into intense, ongoing pain. It may also result in an intense and prolonged painful reaction to normal stimuli, for example, light touch. Over time, the nervous system may "rewire" itself to expect and repeat these strong signals, which is why children with channelopathies after Long COVID can experience chronic, persistent pain that feels out of proportion to any visible injury.

TRPM3 Channels: The Body's Tiny Sensors

One compelling study found that patients with post-COVID-19 condition (i.e., Long COVID) share a significant impairment in something called TRPM3 ion channel activity—a channel also previously shown to be dysfunctional in patients with myalgic encephalomyelitis/chronic fatigue syndrome (ME/CFS). This was observed specifically in natural killer (NK) cells and supports a shared mechanism between Long COVID and ME/CFS. Importantly, both groups demonstrated similarly reduced TRPM3 currents compared to healthy controls. (15)

TRPM3 channels are a type of ion channel that are like tiny "garage doors" on the surface of cells. Their main job is to let calcium ions flow into the cell when needed. Calcium is like a messenger that tells the cell how to react, whether that's activating the immune system, sending nerve signals, or helping muscles work properly.

You can think of TRPM3 channels like a sensor that detects heat, pain, or stress signals. When they open correctly, your body knows how to respond to changes in your environment. But if TRPM3 channels don't work properly, the "sensor" gets confused: signals can be too strong, too weak, or misdirected. This may explain some of the chronic pain, fatigue, or nerve problems people experience after COVID, because the cells aren't receiving or sending messages normally.

Researchers are still studying how channelopathies connect to Long COVID in children, but understanding which "garage doors" are malfunctioning is helping to guide treatment. Future therapies may focus on stabilizing specific ion channels; repairing the doors, tuning down the volume on overactive pain signals, or strengthening weak communication between cells.

In our clinic, we use several technologies and techniques with the goal of normalizing channelopathies.

By understanding and addressing autonomic nervous system dysfunction, we can help children with Long COVID regain their health, energy, and well-being. Instead of merely managing symptoms, we must focus on resetting the body's natural healing mechanisms—starting with the vagus nerve.

Chapter 6:
Centralized Sensitization /
Pain and Inflammation

"Chronic pain is not all about the body, and it's not all about the brain—it's everything. Target everything. Take back your life."

Sean Mackey, MD, PhD

"A spark neglected makes a mighty fire."

Robert Herrick

One of the most misunderstood and frustrating symptoms of Long COVID in children is neuropathic pain, also known as central sensitization. This type of pain is directly linked to inflammation, but it doesn't always show up right away. Instead, it can develop **months** after the initial COVID-19 infection.

Studies have found that the time between the first COVID-19 infection and the onset of neuropathic pain ranges from one month to 15 months (1). Another study showed that half of hospitalized Long COVID patients reported new pain just four weeks after being discharged (2). The pain isn't limited to one area—it can show up anywhere: feet, knees, legs, abdomen, shoulders, hands, back, face, or even the scalp. Some children experience full-body pain, while others feel burning, tingling, electric shock-like pain, itching, or painful cold sensations. Some even lose sensation entirely in certain areas.

Unlike pain from a broken bone or a cut, neuropathic pain is invisible, making it hard for both kids and parents to understand. We've been trained to believe that pain has a quick fix—a pill, a surgery, a treatment—but with chronic pain, it's not that simple. When pain doesn't have an obvious cause, children often feel isolated, misunderstood, and frustrated. Parents struggle to find solutions while doctors may dismiss their concerns or offer treatments that simply don't work.

Traditional pain treatments aren't cutting it for Long COVID. Opioids aren't the answer—they're dangerously overprescribed, leading to a crisis where 70% of all drug overdoses now involve opioids. Meanwhile, other medical interventions like spinal cord stimulators are proving to be ineffective and risky. Long COVID pain is proving tough to treat, and the medical system isn't keeping up.

In contrast to the unmistakable pain caused by well-recognized diseases or injuries like cancer or a fracture, chronic neuropathic pain remains a puzzle to the mind and psyche. It is even more complicated when one considers that children are often not believed when they complain about pain. Many adults, even medical personnel, cannot help but wonder if children are seeking attention or merely exaggerating when they complain of intense pain. Over time, most parents will believe their children. However, it takes a herculean effort to convince doctors of the same.

Even when we know that pain is real, our conditioning leads us to believe that for every problem, there should be a solution in the form of a pill, a procedure, or a surgery, and the pain should subsequently vanish. Endless pain seems illogical, especially when its cause is imperceptible. This can be extremely isolating for children struggling with unseen pain. It also makes for an unenviable journey for their parents.

Young patients contending with conditions that elude external observation eventually become weary of repeatedly explaining, describing, and justifying their situation. They do not know where to turn for help. Traditional treatments for pain, unfortunately, do not seem to be very effective for chronic pain. Not only are young patients misunderstood, but they are also hurting, with seemingly nowhere to turn for help.

The standard definition of intractable pain is pain that cannot be managed by standard medical care. I always tell my patients that medicine has a ceiling. Sooner or later, they will hit that ceiling. Pain does not have a ceiling. The opioid crisis in the US (and worldwide) is soaring. Seventy percent of all drug overdoses now involve opioids.

Almost half the US population uses at least one prescribed medication. Spinal cord stimulators are the implanted medical device of choice for pain, but their results are usually lukewarm, in our experience, and the data is clear: they are dangerous.

The medical solutions for intractable pain simply aren't working, simply because they aren't getting to the root of the problem. In addition, pain associated with Long COVID is certainly falling into the difficult-to-manage category.

Central Sensitization (Central Pain)

Central sensitization refers to a state where the central nervous system amplifies normal sensory input, interpreting it as pain. WebMD defines central pain in the following way: "Central pain syndrome is characterized by a mixture of pain sensations, the most prominent being a constant burning. The steady burning sensation is sometimes increased by light touch. Pain also increases in the presence of temperature changes, most often cold temperatures. A loss of sensation can occur in affected areas, most prominently on distant parts of the body, such as the hands and feet. There may be brief, intolerable bursts of sharp pain on occasion."

It is my hypothesis that neuropathic pain in children associated with Long COVID is a product of pathology stemming from neuroinflammation and other changes resulting from central sensitization and autonomic nervous system dysfunction. It involves two major systems in the body: the nervous system and the immune system. Bear with me as I explain an incredibly complicated cascade of events as simply as possible.

The Role of Histamines in Long COVID and Chronic Pain

Mast cells release histamines. In the last two decades, there has been a particular increase in evidence to support the involvement of H_3 and H_4 receptors in the modulation of neuropathic pain. In the peripheral nervous system, histamine is released in response to tissue injury and/or damage. Through the sensitization of nociceptors (sensory receptors for painful stimuli), histamine may cause increased firing rates, contributing to pain hypersensitivity. In neuropathic pain, histamine released in the periphery by mast cells has been shown to play an important role in the development of hypersensitivity following nerve injury.

Cytokines

Please note: The following sections are quite technical, despite my best efforts. If you are a person who cares less about the details and more about the bottom line, all you need to know is the following:

SARS-CoV-2 affects various players of the child's nervous system and immune system in negative ways, resulting in ongoing inflammation and neurologic damage. This, in turn, may cause future conditions, such as dementia. The rest, you are welcome to skip over. For those of you who want to understand the details, let's delve in!

As previously touched on, cytokines are essential small proteins that play a crucial role in regulating the growth and activity of specific immune and blood cells in children's bodies. They serve as signal carriers to instruct the immune system to carry out its functions. Cytokines exert influence on the growth of various blood cells and other cells involved in the body's immune and inflammatory responses, making them key players in the defense against invaders or perceived threats.

Research has revealed that certain cytokines not only initiate but also sustain pathological (abnormal) pain by directly activating nociceptive sensory neurons. Nociceptors are nerves that detect and respond to damaged parts of the body, such as the pain experienced after a burn.

Inflammatory cytokines are also implicated in nerve injuries and inflammation-induced central sensitization.

In the dorsal root ganglion (DRG), a cluster of afferent sensory nerves located just outside the spinal cord, specific inflammatory cytokines are associated with abnormal pain behaviors and spontaneous activity in injured nerve fibers or neurons.

Multiple studies have demonstrated that both mild and severe cases of COVID-19 can trigger a hyper-inflammatory response, marked by increased levels of various cytokines, including IL-6, IL-8, and TNF-α (3,4).

- **IL-6** plays a central role in the cytokine storm. It is a multi-function cytokine with both anti-inflammatory and pro-inflammatory effects.

- **Interleukin-8 (IL-8)** attracts and activates neutrophils and NK-cells in inflammatory regions. Neutrophils are specialized immune cells that are usually the first immune cells to be dispersed to the site(s) of infection(s). They are capable of preventing viral replication and fighting off other organisms, too.

- **Tumor Necrosis Factor alpha (TNF-α)** is a protein made by the body and a major player in the inflammatory response. It functions by initiating and promoting inflammation. If there is an excess of TNF (or if its presence persists beyond the point where it is needed), it can lead to chronic inflammation.

Although the induction of proinflammatory cytokines is a typical response to viral infection, SARS-CoV-2 has the ability to encode specific proteins that evade the initial type I interferon response (5). This evasion mechanism leads to a prolonged and, in some instances, dysregulated cytokine response.

- **Type I interferons (IFNs)** are released by infected cells, serving three key functions: Firstly, they restrict the spread of infectious agents, particularly viruses. Secondly, they finely tune innate immune responses by promoting certain cell functions while also limiting pro-inflammatory pathways and cytokine production. Thirdly, they play an important role in activating the immune system and helping it to remember specific pathogens in order to make the immune system more effective the next time the body is exposed to the same pathogen.

Various blood panel tests are available for assessing cytokine levels in the body, with a notable focus on their role in conditions like cytokine storms observed in Covid infections. The ELISA panel remains a widely recognized standard for cytokine testing.

When Cytokine Signaling Goes Wrong

Cytokine signaling can trigger a cascade of glial activation and cytokine release within the young brain. Remarkably, even minor infections or sources of inflammation can set off this response in children, circumventing the protective barrier of the BBB.

Glial cells are the immune cells of the brain, functioning as guardians to protect it from injury and disease. These specialized cells play a crucial role in monitoring the pediatric brain's environment and identifying abnormalities.

When microglia detect that something has gone awry, they initiate a response aimed at removing toxic agents and clearing away dead cells. In this way, microglia act as the brain's protectors, actively contributing to the maintenance of a healthy and functioning neural environment in children. Their surveillance and response mechanisms are vital for the overall well-being of the immature central nervous system. These cells, positioned at the intersection of the nervous and immune systems, play a crucial role in this process. The principal glial cells in the central nervous system are microglia, which function as macrophages capable of detecting proinflammatory cytokines.

Upon detecting pro-inflammatory substances like cytokines, microglia respond by producing their own chemicals and additional proinflammatory cytokines. This activation causes the surrounding glial cells to become "excited" or activated. Recent insights indicate that factors such as injury and environmental stressors can lead microglial cells to become 'stuck' in a hyper-excited defensive mode, akin to soldiers constantly on alert for a fight.

Once in this state, even the slightest stimuli can prompt the glial cells to release proinflammatory cytokines, leading to an abnormal pain response in children. This intricate interplay underscores the connection between peripheral inflammation, cytokine signaling, and the modulation of pain responses within the central nervous system.

Toll-like Receptors (TLRs)

Toll-like receptors (TLRs) are an important family of receptors that form the first line of defense system against microbes. They can recognize both pathogens and chemicals released from damaged tissues and dying cells. These receptors can also recognize abnormal patterns associated with the immune response. TLRs form a vital bridge, or link, between the body's immune and nervous systems. TLRs initiate the inflammatory response in an effort to protect the body.

At least one study showed that mice developed allodynia as a response to up-regulation of activation transcription factor 3 (ATF3) in the dorsal root ganglion (DRG). ATF3 is activated by TLRs *(Park, Stokes, Corr & Yaksh, 2014)*. This may explain why so many patients develop allodynia after a COVID-19 infection.

Accumulating evidence now exists showing that TLR activation and its effect on the glial cells and sensory neurons can affect the way humans process pain and lead to states of unresolved and exaggerated pain. Some scientists have been able to reverse nerve pain in rats by administering TLR inhibitors *(Lacagnina, Watkins & Grace, 2018)*.

While all of this may seem complicated, the main takeaway I want you to get from this is that a COVID-19 infection may cause chronic and debilitating pain in children and that the immune system is just as involved in the development of pain as the nervous system. The affected child's body is doing the right thing and fighting valiantly, it's just doing it at the wrong time, and too excessively.

Types of Glial Cells and the Role They Play in Long COVID

In order to understand the big picture, you also have to understand who all the players are, what their roles are, and how they are affected by COVID-19.

Microglia

It has been shown that microglia are significantly reduced in length and number by COVID-19 infections (6). Microglia serve as the child's brain's immune cells, functioning as its protectors against injury and disease. Microglia cells make up 5-10% of the total brain cells. Essentially, microglia act as guardians of the brain's well-being, swiftly responding to pathological invasion.

Recent research indicates that microglia also play a significant role in the developing brain. During this process, more synapses are created than necessary, and only the strongest and most important ones are retained. Microglia directly contribute to this synaptic 'pruning' process by eliminating synapses tagged as unnecessary. Thus, microglia not only act as protectors in the mature brain but also contribute to the sculpting and refinement of neural connections during development.

In neurodegenerative disorders such as Alzheimer's disease, however, the role of microglia may shift. Evidence suggests that microglia can become hyperactivated, promoting neuroinflammation, which may contribute to the formation of characteristic toxic protein deposits like amyloid plaques and neurofibrillary tangles observed in Alzheimer's.

There is a growing hypothesis that Long COVID may be linked to the development of Alzheimer's (a terrifying prospect, if one considers the sheer number of people who are now suffering from Long COVID). Researchers of one study found that having COVID-19 drastically accelerated the structural and functional brain deterioration of patients with dementia, regardless of the type of dementia being experienced (7).

One 2023 study examined neuroinflammatory changes in patients with persistent depressive and cognitive symptoms after COVID-19 infection. This study found that increased microglial activation reveals a possible mechanism to explain persistent depressive cognitive symptoms after the infection (8).

Microglial hyperactivity can continue well after the initial immune response, resulting in long-lasting effects within the central nervous system (CNS). This prolonged reactivity is associated with the up-regulation of proinflammatory cytokine genes, shifts in brain neurochemistry, and a decrease in the growth and development of nerve tissue.

Collectively, these processes can contribute to microglial deterioration, dystrophy, or dysfunction within the CNS, with catastrophic results.

Macroglia

- **Astrocytes**

Astrocytes are characterized by their star-shaped appearance and play a crucial role in maintaining the optimal working environment for neurons. They achieve this by regulating neurotransmitter levels around synapses, controlling concentrations of essential ions such as potassium, and providing metabolic support to neurons.

However, the role of astrocytes extends beyond the mere maintenance of the synaptic environment. Ongoing research delves into how astrocytes actively modulate neuronal communication. Due to their ability to sense neurotransmitter levels in synapses, astrocytes can respond by releasing molecules that directly influence neuronal activity. This capacity positions astrocytes as significant contributors to the modification of synaptic function, highlighting their intricate involvement in shaping the communication between neurons.

One study has found that SARS-CoV-2 has the ability to specifically infect brain astrocytes. This infection is associated with heightened inflammation and neuronal death in the impacted regions of the brain. The research further highlights that SARS-CoV-2, in fact, exhibits a *preference* for infecting astrocytes, where it replicates and propagates, particularly in those astrocytes situated adjacent to infected vasculature.

This finding underscores the complex interaction between the virus and specific cell types within the brain, shedding light on potential neurological effects observed in COVID-19 patients (9).

- **Ependymal Cells**

Ependymal cells are specialized cells that line the spinal cord's central canal and the ventricles of the brain. One of their primary functions is the production and regulation of cerebrospinal fluid (CSF).

Cerebrospinal fluid is a clear, colorless fluid that surrounds the brain and spinal cord, providing mechanical support, buoyancy, and protection to these vital structures. Ependymal cells play a crucial role in maintaining the balance and production of cerebrospinal fluid, contributing to the overall homeostasis of the central nervous system.

Studies conducted on postmortem brains of individuals with COVID-19 have observed the presence of SARS-CoV-2-related transcripts specifically in choroid plexus (CP) epithelial cells and ependymal cells lining the ventricles of the brain. This indicates that the virus may have the ability to infect and impact these specific cell types within the central nervous system (10).

- **Oligodendrocytes**

Oligodendrocytes play a crucial role in providing support to the axons of neurons in the central nervous system, particularly those that traverse long distances within the brain.

These specialized cells produce a fatty substance known as myelin, which forms a protective sheath around axons, serving as insulation. Comparable to the insulation layers around power cables, the myelin sheath facilitates faster transmission of electrical messages along the axons. This insulating property is reflected in the term "white matter," as the white color is attributed to the myelin wrapping around axons.

As a result of hyperimmune responses, COVID-19 has been shown to cause a loss of the myelin sheath around neurons (11). This demyelination process disrupts the normal transmission of electrical signals along the axons, leading to various neurological symptoms and impairments associated with the disease.

In addition, COVID-19 has been shown to reduce the number of oligodendrocytes (12). The oligodendrocytes that do survive the initial infection seem to induce a prolonged inflammatory response (13).

- **Radial cells**

Radial glial cells are a type of progenitor cell with remarkable multipotency, meaning they have the ability to differentiate into various cell types in the nervous system. These cells are particularly notable during early brain development. Radial glial cells serve as a scaffold for migrating neurons, guiding them to their appropriate locations in the developing brain. Additionally, they have the capacity to generate different cell types, including neurons, astrocytes, and oligodendrocytes.

As the nervous system matures, radial glial cells can transition into other cell types, contributing to the formation of the neural network. Their versatility in generating different cell lineages plays a crucial role in the intricate process of brain development and the establishment of its complex structure.

Peripheral glial cells

- **Satellite Cells**

Satellite cells are support cells found in the sensory, sympathetic, and parasympathetic ganglia of the peripheral nervous system. Their primary role is to surround and provide support to neurons within these ganglia. Additionally, satellite cells play a crucial role in regulating the chemical environment around neurons.

Research suggests that satellite cells may contribute to chronic pain. In certain conditions or injuries, satellite cells can become activated and release signaling molecules that influence neuronal function. This activation can lead to changes in the chemical environment, potentially contributing to the development or maintenance of chronic pain states.

Understanding the role of satellite cells in pain modulation is an area of ongoing research and may provide insights into the mechanisms underlying chronic pain conditions.

- **Schwann Cells**

Schwann cells are specialized glial cells that wrap around and myelinate individual axons in the PNS. The myelin sheath they form around axons acts as insulation, enhancing the speed and efficiency of nerve impulse conduction.

While oligodendrocytes in the CNS myelinate multiple axons, each Schwann cell in the PNS typically myelinates a single axon. Both oligodendrocytes and Schwann cells play crucial roles in facilitating the rapid transmission of nerve signals along axons.

One study found that both myelin-making cells (oligodendrocytes or Schwann cells) and neurons are positive for ACE2, indicating that these cells are susceptible to viral attack by SARS-CoV-2.

- **Enteric Glial Cells**

Enteric glial cells are involved in supporting and nourishing neurons in the enteric nervous system. They contribute to the maintenance of the intestinal environment, help modulate the activity of neurons, and participate in the immune responses of the gut. Additionally, enteric glial cells have been implicated in various gastrointestinal disorders and are an active area of research in understanding gut function and dysfunction.

ACE2 has been found throughout the cells of the enteric nervous system, making the enteric nervous system a highly possible entry point into the central nervous system by SARS-CoV-2 (14).

Cytokine Storm

A cytokine storm refers to a hyperinflammatory state that arises due to the uncontrolled and excessive production of cytokines by an overactive and deregulated immune system. This phenomenon can manifest clinically as symptoms such as fever, fatigue, and muscle aches. In severe cases, a cytokine storm can lead to complications like multi-organ failure and abnormal blood clotting, even in children. The most severe instances of a cytokine storm can result in life-threatening conditions and, in some cases, death. This immune system dysregulation is a significant concern in COVID-19 infections.

When people hear about COVID-19, they sometimes worry about something called a "cytokine storm," which is when the body's immune system reacts too strongly all at once during a serious infection. But for many kids with Long COVID, something a little different is happening called Cytokine Release Syndrome, or CRS. This is when the body's immune system stays switched on for a long time and causes ongoing inflammation. It can happen not just with COVID but also with certain medicines or treatments, like chemotherapy or organ transplants.

CRS can make kids feel tired, achy, or feverish, but it can also affect many parts of the body, like the stomach, heart, lungs, kidneys, muscles, and even the brain. That's why kids with Long COVID might have lots of different symptoms that don't seem connected at first—like tummy pain, trouble breathing, headaches, or muscle weakness.

Normally, the immune system sends out messages called cytokines to fight off germs and help the body heal. But with CRS, these messages keep getting sent even when they aren't needed anymore, which is like an army without a leader, causing confusion and damage. This makes it hard for the body to stop being inflamed and to start healing properly. Think of CRS as a wildfire feeding itself. Cytokines stimulate the immune system (15), which then results in further cytokine release.

Knowing about CRS helps us understand why Long COVID can feel so tough and last so long. It shows us that the immune system needs special care to calm down and get back to normal. With the right treatments and support, kids can help their bodies find balance again, reduce inflammation, and start feeling better. This gives hope that recovery is possible, even if it takes time. Your child's body is strong, and with help, it can heal and grow healthy again.

The Effects of Neuroinflammation

Neuroinflammation involves a chronic immune response within the brain characterized by prolonged activation of microglia, the release of inflammatory cytokines, and subsequent oxidative stress. Oxidative stress occurs when there is an imbalance between free radicals and antioxidants in the body.

Both direct and indirect effects of viral infections on the central nervous system (CNS) can initiate neuroinflammation in kids. Infections and trauma within the CNS, as well as in the peripheral nervous system, may both trigger neuroinflammation.

Direct viral effects may include the virus infecting neural cells directly, leading to cellular damage and the activation of the immune response. Indirect effects may involve the systemic immune response to the infection, leading to the release of inflammatory mediators that can affect the brain.

Neuroinflammation can be quite devastating to the developing body. It may lead to a long list of symptoms and effects, including brain fog, fatigue, rapid aging, cancer, autoimmune conditions, pain, blood sugar dysregulation, dysautonomia, cardiac dysfunction, sleep disturbances, hormonal imbalances, fever, memory loss, noise intolerance, psychiatric disorders, and many more. Long-term neuroinflammation may one day lead to neurodegenerative disorders such as Parkinson's, Alzheimer's, and Multiple sclerosis (16).

The dysregulation and prolonged activation of immune cells in the brain, particularly microglia, may result from the lingering effects of the initial viral infection or from ongoing immune responses. This sustained immune activation can lead to persistent inflammation, affecting various aspects of brain function and contributing to the diverse and often fluctuating symptoms reported in pediatric Long COVID cases.

Research in this area is ongoing (although lacking in the pediatric population specifically), and understanding the mechanisms underlying Long COVID is crucial for developing effective strategies for diagnosis, management, and potential treatment of this condition.

Chapter 7:
Depleted Down to the Smallest Cell

"I often wished that more people understood the invisible side of things. Even the people who seemed to understand, didn't really."

Jennifer Starzec

One of the most common complaints of children suffering from Long COVID is down-to-the-bone, all-consuming fatigue. When someone is fatigued, their very life force becomes depleted, making it hard to have the energy to care about anything much more than surviving. Sometimes, even surviving becomes overwhelming. This is especially shocking to parents when it happens to their child, as most children have so much life energy before they fall ill. The contrast can be jarring.

What if this fatigue involves an incredibly complicated domino effect, affecting the very cells that comprise the immune system and the child's body as a whole? Evolving science is pointing to this being the likely scenario.

Mitochondria

Mitochondria, singularly known as mitochondrion, are organelles enclosed by membranes. Mitochondria are often called "the powerhouses of the cell". This description aptly captures their primary function, which is the generation of energy in the form of adenosine triphosphate (ATP). This process, known as oxidative phosphorylation, occurs in the inner mitochondrial membrane and is vital for supplying energy to various cellular activities. Therefore, think of mitochondria as tiny lithium batteries inside our cells, providing the energy for all other cellular functions.

Mitochondria and apoptosis

In addition to energy production, mitochondria play crucial roles in other cellular processes. They are involved in cellular signaling, influencing various aspects of cell function and communication between cells. Mitochondria also have a significant role in regulating cell death through a process called apoptosis. This programmed cell death is essential for maintaining cellular homeostasis, eliminating damaged or unnecessary cells, and plays a key role in various physiological and pathological processes.

Apoptosis refers to the highly regulated and orchestrated process of cell death characterized by specific morphological changes. These changes include membrane DNA fragmentation and cell shrinkage, followed by the swift engulfment of the dying cell by neighboring cells.

While we never think about the fact that in a normal, healthy body, cells need to die when no longer needed, the fact is, humans simply cannot stay alive without this ongoing process of death happening inside the body. This is true even for children. Approximately 10 billion cells undergo programmed cell death every day, serving to balance the constant generation of new cells arising from the body's stem cell populations. This active process ensures the elimination of unwanted or damaged cells, contributing to overall tissue health.

As the body matures and finally ages, the regulation of apoptosis becomes increasingly important. In some cases, apoptotic responses to DNA damage may become less tightly controlled and exaggerated, potentially contributing to degenerative diseases in adulthood. On the other hand, reduced sensitivity in apoptotic responses may contribute to an increased susceptibility to cancer, allowing damaged cells to escape the normal regulatory mechanisms. In order for cancer to develop and grow, apoptosis must be inhibited.

Mitochondria, when healthy, fight cancer. When unhealthy, they fuel cancer. Think of healthy mitochondria as hitmen, specifically targeting cancer (1). Healthy mitochondria are crucial for apoptosis to be performed in the way in which it was designed. If it isn't, it may have devastating consequences to health and well-being. The mitochondria actually fight cancer in ways besides apoptosis, as they regulate many processes that are known to be altered in cancer cells, from metabolism to oxidative stress (2).

How do unhealthy mitochondria help cancer to grow then? It is well-established that defective or dysfunctional mitochondria can contribute to the production of reactive oxygen species (ROS), as mitochondria are a primary source of ROS within the cells, which may lead to cancer developing inside the body. We now know that defective mitochondria are so important when it comes to cancer that cancer literally can't grow without them. Instead of hitmen, unhealthy mitochondria become fuel for cancer (3).

Mitochondria and energy production

Energy production is a central function of mitochondria, their involvement in cellular signaling and apoptosis underscores their importance in maintaining the overall health and functionality of cells.

Simply put, mitochondria produce energy that the body needs to operate. It's how muscles move, how the brain thinks, how the body fights infection and, subsequently, heals. Without the energy from the mitochondria, the body cannot function properly.

In the case of viral infections, they are known to commandeer and destabilize the internal cellular environment, establishing conditions conducive to their own replication. Basically, this virus hijacks the metabolism and then uses that energy to replicate itself instead. It's like an unwanted house guest entering your home and cranking the heat. The virus is clever enough to change the environment to ITS optimal conditions, not the conditions that are best for the host.

The initial SARS-CoV-2 infection is no different and can alter the mitochondria in its host. This can cause cellular energy dysfunction, oxidative stress, and cellular death (4). Muscle tissue has been studied in Long COVID patients which indicated lowered mitochondrial function (5).

Viral proteins have the capability to attach to mitochondrial complexes, leading to disturbances in mitochondrial function and prompting an exaggerated response from immune cells which leads to inflammation. It is also true that the initial COVID-19 virus has the capability to reprogram metabolic systems, as viruses tend to do to replicate and thrive.

It is suspected that, in a person with already low metabolic function and low mitochondrial reserves stemming from preexisting conditions such as diabetes and obesity, the whole system becomes easily overwhelmed by the virus.

Metabolic Reprogramming

We know that the COVID-19 virus changes the way that the body's metabolism functions in different tissues, in order to favor its own replication and ultimately, its own survival. This reprogramming affects many of the building blocks of the body, including the following:

Amino acids

Amino acids are the building blocks of proteins, playing essential roles in various physiological processes, including immune response and cellular function. The intricate relationship between amino acid metabolism and COVID-19 has garnered significant attention in recent studies, shedding light on the potential adverse effects on the body (6).

In the context of COVID-19, there is evidence suggesting a reprogramming of amino acid metabolism during infection. This reprogramming can result in a dysregulation of the delicate balance of amino acids, leading to detrimental consequences. Some studies propose that the virus may manipulate amino acid pathways to facilitate its replication and evade the immune response (7).

One notable aspect is the potential impact on the immune system. Amino acids are crucial for the proper functioning of immune cells, and any disruption in their availability or balance can compromise the immune response against the virus. This dysregulation may contribute to the severity and persistence of COVID-19 symptoms.

Furthermore, alterations in amino acid metabolism may have broader implications for overall cellular health. Amino acids are involved in cellular signaling, energy production, and maintaining cellular structure. Disruptions in these processes can adversely affect various tissues and organs, exacerbating the systemic impact of COVID-19 on the body.

Tryptophan pathways

The impact of COVID-19 on tryptophan pathways has become a subject of interest in understanding the complex interactions between the virus and the host's biochemical processes. Tryptophan, an essential amino acid, is a precursor for various biologically important molecules, including serotonin and kynurenine.

Kynurenine itself is a precursor to several other biologically active compounds, such as kynurenic acid and quinolinic acid. These downstream metabolites have been implicated in various physiological and pathological processes, including immune regulation, neurodegenerative disorders, and inflammation.

Alterations in tryptophan metabolism during COVID-19 may have multifaceted, detrimental effects on both the immune and neurological systems.

One notable aspect is the activation of the enzyme indoleamine 2,3-dioxygenase (IDO), a key player in the tryptophan-kynurenine pathway. Studies suggest that COVID-19 may induce increased IDO activity, leading to a shift in tryptophan metabolism towards the production of kynurenine (8,9). This diversion has been associated with immune modulation, potentially contributing to the observed dysregulation of the immune response in COVID-19 patients.

The consequences of altered tryptophan metabolism extend beyond the immune system. Tryptophan is a precursor for serotonin, a neurotransmitter with crucial roles in mood regulation and mental well-being. Changes in tryptophan availability may influence serotonin synthesis, potentially contributing to neuropsychiatric symptoms reported in individuals affected by COVID-19 (10).

Glutamine

Research on the effects of COVID-19 has revealed intriguing insights into the metabolism of glutamine - an essential amino acid with diverse roles in cellular function.

Glutamine is involved in processes such as energy production, immune function, and the maintenance of cellular integrity. Alterations in glutamine metabolism during COVID-19 may play a significant role in the pathophysiology of COVID-19 infections (11).

One key aspect is the connection between glutamine and the immune response. Glutamine is a crucial nutrient for immune cells, supporting their proliferation and function. In the context of COVID-19, studies suggest that the virus may impact glutamine metabolism, potentially leading to a shift in the availability and utilization of this amino acid by immune cells (11). This alteration in glutamine metabolism could influence the immune system's ability to mount an effective response against the virus.

Furthermore, COVID-19 has been associated with a hyperinflammatory state in children (also called a cytokine storm, discussed in chapter 4 of this book). Glutamine is known for its anti-inflammatory properties, and changes in its metabolism may contribute to the dysregulation of the inflammatory response observed in severe cases of COVID-19. The balance between pro-inflammatory and anti-inflammatory signals is crucial for controlled immune response, and disruptions in glutamine metabolism may tilt this balance.

Moreover, glutamine is a key player in maintaining the integrity of the gastrointestinal tract. COVID-19 has been shown to affect the gastrointestinal system, and alterations in glutamine metabolism could potentially contribute to gastrointestinal symptoms reported by some individuals with the virus.

Arginine reprogramming

Research suggests that COVID-19 may have significant effects on arginine metabolism, a process that involves the essential amino acid arginine (12). Arginine plays a crucial role in various physiological functions, including immune response, vascular health, and the production of nitric oxide. It is a precursor for nitric oxide.

Nitric oxide is a crucial signaling molecule in the body, controlling important functions like vasodilation, immune system, nervous system communication, anti-inflammatory effects, and protecting cells from oxidative stress, to name a few.

COVID-19's potential disruption in arginine metabolism can potentially lead to decreased nitric oxide production. This lowered nitric oxide production may contribute to the vascular complications associated with severe cases of the disease, including endothelial dysfunction and blood clot formation (13). Impaired nitric oxide availability could affect blood vessel function and exacerbate the inflammatory response.

Furthermore, arginine is involved in the regulation of the immune system. It serves as a substrate for the production of various immune-related molecules, and changes in arginine metabolism may influence the immune response to viral infections, including COVID-19. The delicate balance of pro-inflammatory and anti-inflammatory signals in the immune system may be affected by alterations in arginine availability.

As researchers delve deeper into the intricacies of COVID-19 and how it affects children, understanding the effects on arginine metabolism becomes crucial for uncovering potential therapeutic strategies. Targeting arginine pathways may offer avenues for interventions to modulate vascular health, immune response, and overall disease outcomes. Ongoing investigations aim to elucidate the specific mechanisms by which COVID-19 impacts arginine metabolism, providing valuable insights into the complex interplay between the virus and the host's biochemical processes.

Cholesterol

While the exact effects of COVID-19 on cholesterol are unclear at the time of the writing of this book, there is clear evidence that some patients develop diabetes and hyperlipidemia after a COVID-19 infection (14). Cholesterol is a crucial component of cell membranes and serves as a precursor for various molecules, including hormones. The potential impact of COVID-19, particularly Long COVID, on cholesterol metabolism has been a subject of interest.

Some ways in which this may affect the young body include:

- **Inflammatory Response**: COVID-19 can trigger a systemic inflammatory response. Inflammation may influence cholesterol metabolism, potentially leading to alterations in lipid profiles. Persistent inflammation in Long COVID might have implications for cholesterol homeostasis.

- **Organ Damage**: COVID-19 can lead to organ damage, including effects on the liver. The liver plays a central role in cholesterol metabolism. Any disruption in liver function could impact the synthesis, storage, and transportation of cholesterol in the body.

- **Immune System Modulation**: Cholesterol is essential for the proper functioning of immune cells. Changes in cholesterol metabolism might affect the immune response, and considering the immune dysregulation reported in long COVID, there could be connections between the immune system function, inflammation, and cholesterol.

- **Cardiovascular Implications**: Altered cholesterol metabolism is often associated with cardiovascular risk factors. COVID-19 and Long COVID have been linked to cardiovascular complications (15). Understanding the relationship between cholesterol metabolism and cardiovascular health in the context of Long COVID is an area of ongoing investigation.

There is also a very strong possibility that the COVID-19 virus causes the child's body to change the way its own metabolism is functioning, in an effort to rid itself of the virus (16). This means that metabolic reprogramming may be happening on two fronts: the virus may affect your child's metabolism, but it may also be forcing his or her body to affect its own metabolism.

The Weakened Immune System

Long COVID may affect the young immune system in various ways:

- **Persistent Inflammation**: Pediatric Long COVID is often associated with persistent inflammation, indicating ongoing immune system activation. The immune system, in its attempt to fight off the virus during the acute phase, might remain activated, contributing to the prolonged symptoms observed in Long COVID. As discussed in Chapter 4, dysregulated cytokine production – sometimes referred to as a cytokine storm – is associated with severe COVID-19. In Long COVID, there may be a persistent imbalance in cytokine levels, contributing to ongoing symptoms and potentially affecting the immune system in detrimental ways (17).

- **Immune Dysregulation**: Some studies suggest that Long COVID may involve immune dysregulation, where the immune response is imbalanced. This dysregulation may manifest as a prolonged inflammatory state or, in some cases, a compromised ability to fight off other infections (18).

- **Autoimmunity Dysregulation**: Autoimmunity occurs when the immune system mistakenly targets its own cells.

- **Molecular Mimicry:** Molecular mimicry is a phenomenon where viral components resemble the body's own proteins. In the case of Long COVID, it's possible that the immune response, originally directed against the virus, may start targeting similar-looking proteins in the body, leading to autoimmune reactions.

- **Immunological Memory:** The immune system forms a memory of encountered pathogens, including SARS-CoV-2. In some cases, this memory might lead to a prolonged immune response that continues to affect the body's own tissues, contributing to autoimmune-like manifestations.

- **Tissue Damage and Exposure of Self-Antigens**: The initial viral infection and subsequent inflammation in COVID-19 can cause tissue damage. This damage may expose normally hidden self-antigens, prompting the immune system to recognize and attack its own tissues.

- **Impact on Specific Immune Cells**: Long COVID may affect specific immune cells. For example, studies have reported changes in the numbers and function of T cells, B cells, and other immune components (19). These

alterations could contribute to the immune
dysregulation observed in long COVID in children.

Reactivation of Old Viruses

A latent virus refers to a situation where the viral RNA or
DNA persists within the cells of the body following the initial
infection. During this latent phase, these viruses do not actively
replicate or induce disease symptoms. However, despite their
dormancy, latent viruses have the potential to be transmissible
to others. What distinguishes these viruses is their ability to
remain in the body for extended periods, often for an entire
lifetime, without causing noticeable symptoms or recurrent
infections. These infections often start in childhood.

It's important to highlight that certain external factors,
such as stress or the presence of additional viral infections, can
serve as triggers for the reactivation of latent viruses. This
reactivation process involves the resumption of viral replication
and may lead to the recurrence of symptoms or the shedding of
the virus, making it contagious once again.

During viral reactivation, these dormant, latent viruses
switch back on into what is known as the lytic phase. During
this phase, the virus is capable of replication and can cause
symptoms in children. These symptoms can be similar to the
initial viral infection or may develop completely new symptoms
when the virus reactivates. One common example of this is the
varicella-zoster virus that causes chickenpox. During the initial
infection of the virus, a person experiences a chickenpox
infection or varicella. Once the infection passes, the virus
remains in the ganglionic neurons of the body as a latent virus.
When reactivated, this virus triggers herpes zoster, known
more commonly as shingles.

When a child contracts acute COVID-19, there is a notable reduction in his or her T cells. This reduction in T cells creates an environment where latent viruses, such as Epstein-Barr Virus (EBV), can be reactivated. Normally, T cells play a crucial role in keeping these latent viruses under control.

The reactivation of latent viruses, triggered by the SARS-CoV-2 virus during acute COVID-19, can result in these viruses entering an active state and causing symptoms. Long COVID has been associated with the reactivation of latent viruses (20). This phenomenon has been particularly noted in patients experiencing severe and debilitating fatigue, a common symptom in Long COVID. In some cases, this fatigue is severe enough to lead to a comorbid diagnosis of Myalgic Encephalomyelitis/Chronic Fatigue Syndrome (ME/CFS).

Researchers have focused on understanding the connection between Long COVID and Epstein-Barr Virus (EBV), a herpes virus known to be associated with ME/CFS. Recent studies in this area have found that a significant proportion of individuals with Long COVID (66.7% in one study) (21) tested positive for EBV reactivation. This suggests a potential link between the reactivation of EBV and the persistent symptoms observed in Long COVID, emphasizing the complex interplay between viral infections and the immune system in the context of post-acute sequelae of SARS-CoV-2 infection.

The Possible Long-Term Toll of Long COVID:

Cancer

Earlier in this chapter, I discussed the role that the COVID-19 virus plays in interfering with mitochondrial function. As mentioned, the mitochondria play a crucial role in the body's ability to fight cancer. So does inflammation. It is common knowledge that chronic inflammation may lead to DNA damage and eventually, cancer. However, COVID-19 and Long COVID may cause cancer in other ways, too.

There are at least seven viruses known to cause cancer in humans. These are called oncogenic viruses, and include the human papillomavirus (HPV), the Epstein-Barr Virus (EBV), and the human T-cell leukemia virus I (HTLV-1), to name a few. Therefore, the idea that a virus may cause cancer is not just a theory, but a fact.

The characteristics of SARS-CoV-2 and its inflammatory features suggest a resemblance to oncogenic viruses. However, it's important to note that as of now, there is no direct evidence or long-term observation supporting the hypothesis that SARS-CoV-2 acts as an oncogenic virus. While the virus shares some characteristics with viruses known to contribute to cancer development, more research and time are needed to establish any direct link between SARS-CoV-2 infection and the induction of cancer.

The long-term effects of SARS-CoV-2 infection are a cause for concern, particularly in relation to the potential development of malignant neoplasms, which are cancerous growths. This could become a significant health issue in the years to come. The infection influences various mechanisms that are vital in the initiation and progression of cancer, including the regulation of the cell cycle, and pathways related to inflammation, destruction of old or damaged cells, and cell proliferation.

These disruptions in cellular processes may contribute to an increased risk of cancer, highlighting the importance of understanding and monitoring the potential long-term consequences of COVID-19.

A report from the Centers for Disease Control and Prevention (CDC) in December 2022 revealed an increase in the annual number of cancer deaths from 2018 to 2021 (22). This increase of 4.7% comes after a prolonged period of declining cancer mortality.

The report suggests that the rise in cancer deaths is not solely attributed to a decrease in screening, but there are disproportionate increases in cancer deaths linked to COVID-19 as an underlying cause. The increase is noted to be higher among males, members of ethnic or racial minority groups, and individuals with specific types of cancers such as lymphoma, leukemia, or myeloma.

Doctors all over the world are reporting an increase in individuals seeking help for cancers such as breast, prostate, pancreatic, and colorectal.

One such oncologist, Dr. Kashyap Patel, reported a strange uptick in very aggressive cancers, as well as cancers now affecting individuals 20-30 years earlier than the typical presentation (23).

Currently, there is no definitive evidence indicating an overall increase in childhood leukemia. That being said, no long-term studies have been done on this specific subject. Some researchers have proposed a "delayed reaction" hypothesis. This hypothesis basically proposes that the immune system needs training and practice in order to function perfectly. This "training" often occurs in early childhood, when children are exposed to early childhood diseases by interacting with other kids. The "delayed infection" hypothesis suggests that if this exposure did not happen because of limited social interaction during COVID, it could lead to an increase in leukemia rates at a later stage.

Another hypothesis studied mainly by Greaves is regarding acute lymphoblastic leukemia (ALL), a major subtype of pediatric cancer (24). It states that in order for ALL to be triggered, there are two distinct steps: the first one happens in utero, by a process called fusion gene formation. In a nutshell, this means that the baby's genome is structurally rearranged, which can lead to two previously separated genes being in close proximity and eventually fusing to form a hybrid gene. Later on, in a small number of cases, a secondary negative event (such as a viral infection) causes another genetic change and ultimately results in the development of ALL. Again, the theory holds that exposure to microbes early in life "trains" the immune system correctly. In the absence of this training process, later exposure to microbes triggers later infections to result in secondary adverse gene mutations. It is possible that the combination of quarantine and infection may result in an increase in childhood leukemia cases, but only time will tell.

Dementia

Findings from a small study supported by the National Institute of Neurological Disorders and Stroke (NINDS) highlight the concerning impact of COVID-19 on individuals with dementia (25). The study focused on the cognitive effects of COVID-19 in people already diagnosed with dementia and revealed that the virus led to a rapid acceleration of both structural and functional brain deterioration, regardless of the type of dementia.

During the Alzheimer's Association International Conference, a researcher from The University of Texas Health Science Center at San Antonio shared findings from a study involving over 400 older adults in Argentina who had recovered from COVID-19. The results indicated that over 60% of these individuals exhibited some level of cognitive impairment.

Dr. de Erausquin and a team of researchers are conducting the study in collaboration with the Cognitive Neuropsychiatric Sequelae of SARS-CoV-2 (CNS SC2) consortium, a global initiative led by the Alzheimer's Association. This study is ongoing, and individuals will be followed up with over the next 3-5 years. At this time, it is not known if the cognitive dysfunction will be permanent or progressive.

In the Argentine participant group, 78% had a confirmed recovery from SARS-CoV-2 infection through polymerase chain reaction (PCR) testing, while the remaining quarter of volunteers never contracted the virus.

Among the 60% of individuals who had recovered from COVID-19 and displayed cognitive impairment, approximately one in three exhibited severe cognitive impairment resembling a "dementia-like syndrome". This syndrome shares similarities with dementia, but may not be persistent or progressive.

Dr. de Erausquin expressed concern about the findings, noting that people in the 60 to 70 age range typically have a 6% lifetime risk of developing Alzheimer's disease. However, the Argentine study population showed a cognitive impairment rate that is 10 times higher, raising worries about the potential for a dementia-related epidemic linked to the latest coronavirus.

Persistent loss of smell, a common symptom of COVID-19, seems to also be associated with changes in the brain and long-term cognitive dysfunction. The olfactory bulb, housing the brain cells responsible for processing smells, is a key entry point for the virus into the nervous system. This highlights a potential link between the neurological impact of COVID-19 and the manifestation of symptoms such as anosmia (loss of smell).

While the data is not definitive yet, I have personally had a patient who, at the age of 50, experienced a sudden onset of frontal lobe dementia and became non-verbal within two weeks of contracting COVID-19. Within months, she was exposed a second time and passed away within a week. The speed at which this patient deteriorated astounded my team and her family.

I think it is highly probable that over the following years, we will see an explosion of dementia cases, as well as dementia onset at a young age. All the conditions that make the brain fertile for the development of dementia seem to be brought about by this virus.

While we may not yet fully understand the role that long COVID plays in the human body, it is clear that it has devastating effects on the body's systems, organs, and cells, down to the smallest building blocks that make up the body. It is clear that both acute and long COVID may cause long-term and even life-threatening complications that I am certain will be revealed over time.

Chapter 8:
How do I help my child?
(Supplements and therapies)

"It does not matter how slowly you go so long as you do not stop."

Confucius

"Adopt the pace of nature: her secret is patience."

Ralph Waldo Emerson

In chapter 10, I'll share the core program we've developed to help children recover from long COVID. It's a powerful, intensive protocol that we've seen work with extraordinary results. However, it comes with challenges: it's not typically covered by insurance, it requires a major time commitment—four days a week for several months—and temporary relocation to Arkansas, which simply isn't feasible for many families.

So what do you do when a program like this is out of your reach?

What do you do when you've already taken your child to countless doctors with no answers, and "just accepting it" isn't an option?

You fight.

You fight for your child in the most intelligent, committed, and relentless way possible. That means becoming the architect of their care plan. You'll need to research—carefully, deeply, and consistently. You'll need to identify therapies available locally and pair them with supplements supported by emerging evidence. You'll need to build a plan that's both practical and powerful. You will need help.

And most of all, you'll need to be patient.

Healing isn't a straight line—it's a winding river that moves at its own pace. Some days you'll feel progress; others may feel like setbacks. That's normal. There are no straight rivers. What matters is staying the course.

Track everything.

Keep a daily log or symptom journal. Rate your child's top symptoms on a scale of 0 to 10. If they're old enough, let them participate. This builds self-awareness and gives you clear data over time. Patterns will emerge. You'll begin to see what's working—and what's not. Do not be attached to the numbers, do not allow the numbers to affect you or your child emotionally. It is merely data, and you are simply collecting it.

Resist the urge to change things too quickly. Healing takes time, and pulling the plug on therapy too early may rob you of answers. Be systematic. Give each strategy time to prove itself.

Above all, don't carry the weight of your child's healing on your shoulders.

You are not expected to know everything. You are expected to try. Every decision, every attempt, every step forward (even the ones that don't work) is part of the process. Ruling something in—or out—is still progress.

Every single child I've seen recover shares one thing in common: A caregiver who refused to give up. Be that person. You may succeed or you may not, but one day you will know that you did everything you could have. You have little to lose and everything to gain.

Things you can do or take at home:

IgG Food Sensitivity Testing:

Why it's helpful:

When dealing with digestive challenges—especially in the context of chronic illness—pinpointing which foods your body reacts to can be a game-changer. While there's a fair amount of controversy surrounding food sensitivity testing, particularly IgG testing, I've found it to be a consistently valuable tool in clinical practice. Despite some healthcare professionals dismissing it as unreliable, my experience treating hundreds of complex patients tells a different story.

Much of the debate stems from traditional medical training, which focuses primarily on IgE-mediated allergies—those that cause immediate and often severe reactions like hives, swelling, or anaphylaxis. These types of allergies are rare and usually obvious, as symptoms appear quickly after exposure. Think peanuts or shellfish—you'll know right away if your body can't tolerate them.

IgG testing, by contrast, identifies delayed immune responses to food—reactions that can take up to 72 hours to appear and may not be as clear-cut. These sensitivities can manifest in a wide range of symptoms, from digestive issues and brain fog to joint pain, fatigue, mood swings, and inflammation. This makes them harder to connect to a specific food without testing. Many of our patients rank this test among the most insightful parts of their treatment—giving them clarity on what their body might be quietly reacting to, even when the foods seem healthy or "safe."

The lab we most often recommend for IgG testing is Alletess, primarily because of their reliable results and the convenience of their at-home finger-prick kit. That said, many labs offer similar tests, and some may be more affordable. It's important to note, however, that the test has limitations. It's only effective if the patient has been regularly consuming a diverse range of foods. If someone has been avoiding certain items for an extended period (say, gluten for several years), their immune system may no longer produce detectable antibodies to those foods, leading to a misleading "safe" result.

Important:

Ultimately, IgG testing isn't a magic bullet—it's a starting point. It should be used in conjunction with symptom tracking and personal insight, not as a replacement for clinical judgment or lived experience.

Simple Spectrum ®

Why It Is Helpful:

Simple Spectrum® is a comprehensive, high-quality nutritional supplement formulated specifically for children with neurological and developmental challenges, and it may offer valuable support for pediatric Long COVID recovery. The product includes therapeutic doses of methylated B vitamins (B6, B12, and folate), minerals (zinc, magnesium, selenium), antioxidants (CoQ10, NAC), and other nutrients essential for mitochondrial function, immune regulation, and cognitive health. These components are particularly relevant in pediatric Long COVID, where symptoms such as fatigue, brain fog, anxiety, and dysregulation of the nervous and immune systems are common. The use of bioavailable (methylated and chelated) forms supports children who may have MTHFR mutations or absorption issues, reducing the burden on detox and methylation pathways. While not studied specifically in Long COVID, the formula aligns with emerging integrative approaches aimed at restoring function in children with chronic post-viral conditions. By providing foundational nutritional support in one well-tolerated product, Simple Spectrum may serve as a convenient and strategic part of a broader pediatric Long COVID care plan. Order at www.simplespectrumsupplement.com

Important

- **IF YOU CAN ONLY AFFORD ONE SUPPLEMENT, THIS SHOULD BE YOUR GO-TO!**

- Uses therapeutic doses based on clinical research, not just RDAs

- Includes methylated forms of B vitamins, which support detox and methylation

- Contains no artificial colors, sweeteners, or preservatives

- Designed to be neurologically supportive, which is especially relevant for symptoms like brain fog, anxiety, and fatigue seen in Long COVID

- Convenient all-in-one formula reduces supplement burden for kids and caregivers

Dosage

- Children under 6 years: typically ½ scoop daily, mixed with food or drink

- Children 6 and older: typically 1 scoop daily

- Always begin with a lower dose and increase gradually to monitor tolerance

- Should be taken with food for best absorption and to reduce the chance of mild nausea

Probiotics and Gut Support

Why it's helpful:

Children recovering from long COVID often experience disruptions in their gut microbiome, including a decrease in beneficial bacteria like Bifidobacterium. This imbalance can contribute to lingering symptoms such as digestive issues, fatigue, and mood disturbances.

To support gut health, incorporating both probiotics and prebiotics into a child's diet can be beneficial. Probiotics are live beneficial bacteria found in certain foods and supplements, while prebiotics are dietary fibers that feed these good bacteria. For instance, glucomannan, a soluble fiber derived from konjac root, has been shown to promote the growth of beneficial gut bacteria and improve digestive health. Similarly, chia seeds provide both soluble and insoluble fiber, supporting a healthy gut environment.

A product like ION* Gut Support by Intelligence of Nature offers a mineral-based supplement aimed at strengthening the gut lining and supporting the microbiome. It's important to choose products that are free from added sugars, gluten, casein, and soy to avoid potential inflammatory responses.

Important:

Caution is advised when introducing prebiotics, especially if a child has conditions like small intestinal bacterial overgrowth (SIBO), as prebiotics can sometimes exacerbate symptoms by feeding harmful bacteria. In such cases, focusing on probiotics and fermented foods may be more appropriate. Always consult with a pediatric healthcare provider before starting any new supplement regimen to ensure it's suitable for your child's specific health needs.

Enzyme Therapy (Nattokinase)

Why it's helpful:

Nattokinase, an enzyme derived from the Japanese fermented soybean dish *natto*, has gained attention for its potential role in managing long COVID symptoms, primarily due to its fibrinolytic (clot-dissolving) properties. Preliminary studies in adults suggest that nattokinase may help degrade fibrin and possibly even the SARS-CoV-2 spike protein, which has been implicated in persistent symptoms associated with long COVID. These findings are largely based on in vitro experiments and anecdotal patient reports, with no large-scale clinical trials confirming its efficacy or safety.

Important:

Despite growing interest, there is currently no research supporting the use of nattokinase for long COVID in pediatric patients. As such, its use in children should be approached with caution and only under the guidance of a qualified healthcare provider, especially considering the absence of age-specific dosing guidelines and potential interactions with other treatments.

Melatonin

Why It's Helpful:

Melatonin, a hormone naturally produced by the body, is renowned for regulating sleep-wake cycles. Beyond its role in sleep, melatonin exhibits antioxidant, anti-inflammatory, and immunomodulatory properties, which may be beneficial in managing Long COVID symptoms. In adults, melatonin has been suggested to alleviate cognitive issues like "brain fog," chronic fatigue, and muscle weakness associated with Long COVID. Its anti-inflammatory action involves mechanisms such as the suppression of nuclear factor-kappa B (NF-κB) activation and the reduction of pro-inflammatory cytokines like IL-6 and TNF-α. Additionally, melatonin's antioxidant effects help mitigate oxidative stress, potentially protecting against mitochondrial dysfunction observed in Long COVID patients. While direct studies on melatonin's efficacy in pediatric Long COVID are limited, its established safety profile and multifaceted benefits make it a candidate for symptom management in children (1).

Important:

- **Safety Profile:** Melatonin is generally considered safe for short-term use in children.

- **Medical Supervision:** Always consult a healthcare provider before initiating melatonin, especially for children with underlying health conditions or those taking other medications.

- **Potential Side Effects:** Some children may experience side effects such as morning drowsiness, headaches, or increased bedwetting.

- **Long-Term Use:** The long-term effects of melatonin use in children are not well-studied; therefore, ongoing evaluation by a healthcare provider is recommended.

Dosing Guidelines:

- **Starting Dose:** Begin with 0.5 to 1 mg at bedtime.

- **Formulation:** Slow-release formulations are preferred to mimic the body's natural melatonin secretion and support sustained sleep.

- **Titration:** If well-tolerated, the dose can be gradually increased.

- **Maximum Dose:** Up to 3–6 mg in older children, based on clinical response and under medical supervision.

BPC-157

Why It's Helpful:

BPC-157, a synthetic peptide derived from a protective protein in the stomach, has garnered attention for its potential therapeutic effects in various conditions. In preclinical studies, BPC-157 has demonstrated the ability to modulate vasomotor tone through the activation of endothelial nitric oxide synthase (eNOS), leading to nitric oxide (NO) release. This mechanism supports vascular integrity and modulates immune responses, which are critical factors in conditions like Long COVID. Additionally, BPC-157 has shown neuroprotective effects in animal models, including the amelioration of concussive brain injuries and the protection of somatosensory neurons. These properties suggest that BPC-157 may offer benefits in addressing the vascular and neurological complications associated with Long COVID (2).

Important:

While BPC-157 shows promise in preclinical studies, it's important to note that human clinical trials are limited, and its safety and efficacy in pediatric populations have not been established. Therefore, its use in children, especially for conditions like Long COVID, should be approached with caution and under the guidance of a qualified healthcare professional. Further research is necessary to determine appropriate dosing, safety profiles, and therapeutic efficacy in both adults and children.

Vitamins D3 and K2

Why It's Helpful:

Vitamin D3 supports the immune system by modulating the activity of immune cells and reducing the production of pro-inflammatory cytokines. This action may alleviate persistent inflammation associated with Long COVID. Vitamin K2 complements this by activating proteins that regulate calcium deposition, thereby preventing vascular calcification and supporting cardiovascular health. Together, these vitamins may help mitigate some of the vascular and inflammatory complications observed in Long COVID. While more research is needed, especially in pediatric populations, the synergistic effects of Vitamins D3 and K2 present a promising avenue for supporting recovery from Long COVID symptoms.

Vitamin D3 (cholecalciferol) is known for its immunomodulatory and neuroprotective properties, while Vitamin K2 (particularly the MK-7 form) activates proteins that support bone mineralization and inhibit vascular stiffness. A study published in *Nutrients* demonstrated that supplementation with Vitamins D3 and K2 improved the Long COVID Index and reduced several inflammatory markers in adults (3). While direct studies in children are limited, these findings suggest potential benefits for pediatric populations experiencing Long COVID symptoms.

Important:

Vitamin K2 supplementation in children is less clearly defined; however, ensuring adequate intake through diet or supplements may support bone and cardiovascular health. It's crucial to consult a healthcare provider before starting any new supplement regimen, especially for children.

Dosage:

For children, the recommended daily intake of Vitamin D varies by age:

- Infants (0–12 months): 400 IU (10 mcg)
- Children (1 year and older): 600 IU (15 mcg)

Magnesium

How It May Help:

Magnesium is a vital mineral involved in over 300 biochemical reactions in the body, including nerve function, muscle contraction, and immune regulation. In the context of pediatric Long COVID, magnesium deficiency has been associated with symptoms such as fatigue, brain fog, headaches, dizziness, and muscle pain. A study highlighted that children consuming less than 75% of their recommended dietary allowance (RDA) for magnesium exhibited elevated serum C-reactive protein (CRP) levels, indicating increased inflammation. Furthermore, magnesium plays a role in modulating the immune response and reducing oxidative stress, which are crucial factors in the pathophysiology of Long COVID (4).

Important:

- While magnesium supplementation may offer benefits, it's essential to approach it cautiously. Excessive intake can lead to side effects such as diarrhea, nausea, and abdominal cramping.

- Children with kidney disorders should avoid magnesium supplements unless prescribed by a healthcare provider, as impaired kidney function can lead to magnesium accumulation and toxicity.

- It's also important to consider potential interactions with other medications the child may be taking. Therefore, always consult with a pediatrician or healthcare professional before initiating magnesium supplementation.

- Not all forms of magnesium are equally suited for every child. Some types may worsen diarrhea, while others are more effective for calming the nervous system, improving sleep, or reducing muscle pain. Choosing the right form depends on the child's specific symptoms and medical condition.

Magnesium Forms for Pediatric Long COVID

Symptom/Condition	Best Magnesium Form(s)	Forms to Avoid
Chronic diarrhea / Irritable Bowel Syndrome	Glycinate, Malate, Taurate	Citrate, Oxide, Hydroxide, Sulfate

Constipation	Citrate, Hydroxide	Glycinate, Malate
Anxiety, insomnia, brain fog	Glycinate, Threonate, Taurate	Oxide, Sulfate
Fatigue, muscle pain, post-exertional malaise	Malate, Glycinate	Oxide, Sulfate
Cardiovascular symptoms (palpitations)	Taurate, Orotate	Oxide, Sulfate
Kidney disease	Only under medical supervision	Most forms (toxicity risk)

Dosage:

The Recommended Dietary Allowances (RDAs) for magnesium in children are as follows :

- Ages 1–3 years: 80 mg/day

- Ages 4–8 years: 130 mg/day

- Ages 9–13 years: 240 mg/day

- For supplementation purposes, a common approach is to administer 9 mg/kg/day of a soluble form of magnesium, such as magnesium glycinate, which is better absorbed

and less likely to cause gastrointestinal side effects.
However, dosing should be individualized based on your
child's specific needs and under medical supervision.

Blue-Green Algae

How It May Help:

Blue-green algae, particularly spirulina, is rich in nutrients
like protein, B vitamins, iron, and antioxidants, which support
immune function and reduce inflammation. These properties
may help alleviate symptoms associated with Long COVID in
children, such as fatigue and cognitive difficulties. Spirulina has
demonstrated antioxidant and anti-inflammatory effects,
potentially aiding in the recovery process. In addition,
Phycocyanin, a blue pigment found in blue-green algae (like
Spirulina), has shown strong anti-inflammatory, antioxidant,
and immune-modulating properties. In pediatric Long
COVID—where symptoms like fatigue, inflammation, brain
fog, and immune dysregulation are common—these actions
may offer meaningful support. Phycocyanin helps scavenge free
radicals, reduce oxidative stress, and regulate cytokine
production, which are all disrupted in post-viral syndromes. It
has also been shown to support mitochondrial protection and
improve neuroinflammation, both key concerns in Long
COVID recovery.

Important Considerations

- While spirulina is generally considered safe for children,
  it's crucial to ensure the product is free from
  contaminants like microcystins, which can cause liver
  damage. Children are more sensitive to these toxins, so
  selecting high-quality, tested products is essential.
  Consulting with a holistic or knowledgeable pediatric

healthcare provider before starting supplementation is recommended to ensure safety and appropriate dosing.

- Acts as a **COX-2 inhibitor**, reducing inflammation without the side effects of NSAIDs (5)

- Promotes **glutathione production**, supporting detox and immune balance

- Supports **mitochondrial health**, critical for improving energy and fatigue symptoms

- Natural compound with a strong **safety profile**, especially in food-based forms like Spirulina

Dosage:

Clinical studies have used spirulina in various dosages. For example, an 8-week study administered 2 grams daily to preschool-aged children without adverse effects. However, there are no standardized dosing guidelines for children. Therefore, it's important to consult a healthcare professional to determine the appropriate dosage based on individual needs and health status.

Minerals

How it may help:

Mineral supplements can play a powerful role in helping children recover from Long COVID by supporting energy, immune health, and nervous system function. Kids with Long COVID often face fatigue, brain fog, and inflammation — symptoms that can worsen if key minerals like magnesium, zinc, and selenium are low. These nutrients help fight inflammation, boost energy at the cellular level, and regulate the immune system. Addressing even mild deficiencies may help children bounce back faster and feel more like themselves again.

Important:

- Research shows that minerals like zinc can help modulate immune responses and reduce viral replication.

- Magnesium plays a key role in reducing inflammation and supporting mitochondrial energy production (6).

- Selenium is also vital for antioxidant defense and thyroid function. A review by DiNicolantonio et al. (2021) supports using these minerals to improve outcomes in viral infections, including COVID-19 (7).

Dosage:

- Mineral supplementation should always be guided by a healthcare provider, especially in children. Blood work may reveal specific deficiencies, allowing for targeted treatment. Common starting doses under clinical guidance include:

- **Zinc**: 5–10 mg/day for younger children, up to 20 mg/day for teens

- **Magnesium**: 100–200 mg/day, depending on age and form (e.g., magnesium glycinate for better absorption)

- **Selenium**: 20–40 mcg/day, adjusted based on diet and labs

- Avoid high doses without supervision, as excess intake can be harmful. Food-based sources and a balanced diet should always be the foundation.

- Avoid supplements containing copper, as that may make brain fog worse.

- I recommend CT Minerals® by Cellcore as a high-quality mineral supplement easily absorbed and utilized by the body.

Methylated B Vitamins

Why It May Be Helpful:

Some people (especially children with chronic health conditions like Long COVID) may have trouble converting standard (inactive) forms of B vitamins into their active forms. Methylated B vitamins (especially B9 (methylfolate) and B12 (methylcobalamin)) play a vital role in supporting neurological health, energy production, and detoxification. Methylfolate (also written as L-methylfolate or 5-MTHF) is the active form of folate (vitamin B9) that your body can use immediately, without needing to convert it.

In children with Long COVID, symptoms like fatigue, brain fog, anxiety, and poor focus may be linked to impaired methylation pathways or inflammation in the nervous system. Methylated forms are more readily absorbed and used by the body, especially in individuals with genetic variants like MTHFR. These activated B vitamins may help improve energy, mood, and cognitive clarity—helping kids feel more like themselves again.

Important:

Methylated B vitamins are especially relevant in pediatric Long COVID because they:

- Support mitochondrial energy production, which is impaired in Long COVID.

- Help regulate neurotransmitters like serotonin and dopamine, improving mood and focus.

- Promote healthy homocysteine levels, reducing systemic inflammation (8).

- Are often better tolerated in kids with MTHFR or other methylation issues.

- Bypass genetic and metabolic bottlenecks, making them easier for the body to use immediately — especially in children with impaired methylation or detox pathways.

Always take B12 WITH B6. Failure to do so may lead to imbalances. For example, taking B12 alone in high doses without B6 may lead to neurotransmitter imbalance or under-functioning detox pathways. Taking B6 alone without enough B12 (and folate) may allow toxic buildup of homocysteine or unmetabolized intermediates.

Dosage:

Always consult a healthcare provider for lab testing and appropriate dosing. General pediatric guidance includes:

- **Methylfolate (B9):** 200–400 mcg/day for children; 400–800 mcg/day for teens

- **Methylcobalamin (B12):** 250–500 mcg/day orally or sublingually

- **Combined B-complex (methylated):** Often used 2–5 times per week. Start low and increase gradually, as some children may be sensitive to rapid methylation changes.

- **Pyridoxal-5'-phosphate (PLP or P5P) — (the active form of vitamin B6):** 2–10 mg/day in younger children, and 10–25 mg/day in older children and teens

Manganese

Why It May Be Helpful:

Manganese may offer meaningful support for children affected by Long COVID and hypermobile Ehlers-Danlos syndrome (hEDS) due to its role in both nervous system and connective tissue function. In the context of pediatric Long COVID, manganese activates manganese superoxide dismutase (MnSOD), a crucial antioxidant enzyme that helps defend neurons and mitochondria from oxidative stress—an issue frequently reported in post-viral fatigue and cognitive dysfunction. It also contributes to the production of neurotransmitters like dopamine and glutamate, which influence energy regulation, concentration, and mood, all of which are commonly disrupted in affected children.

For children with hEDS, manganese supports the formation of glycosaminoglycans (GAGs)—molecules critical for the integrity of connective tissue, cartilage, and tendons. Though it doesn't address the underlying genetic collagen defects seen in hEDS, it may assist in improving tissue structure and healing by supporting enzymes involved in collagen turnover. This could be beneficial for joint stability, wound repair, and overall tissue resilience.

Important:

- Manganese is a trace mineral, which means it's required only in very small amounts. Excess intake can be toxic—especially for children.

- Neurological symptoms, such as tremors, irritability, or coordination issues, can occur with high manganese levels due to its tendency to accumulate in the brain.

- Iron deficiency increases manganese absorption, making iron-deficient children more susceptible to manganese overload.

- Manganese can interact with antacids, antibiotics, and laxatives, which may impair absorption or cause imbalances if used together.

Dosage:

Recommended daily intake for children:

- 4–8 years: ~1.2 mg/day

- 9–13 years: ~1.9 mg/day

- 14–18 years:

- Boys: ~2.2 mg/day/Girls: ~1.6 mg/day

Common supplemental doses:

- Typically 0.5–2 mg/day, often found in multivitamin or trace mineral formulas

Manganese is often paired with supportive nutrients like vitamin C, lysine, proline, glutathione, and CoQ10 in integrative protocols to promote tissue repair and antioxidant defense.

N-Acetylcysteine (NAC)

How It May Help:

N-Acetylcysteine (NAC) is a precursor to glutathione, a critical antioxidant that supports immune function and reduces oxidative stress. In pediatric patients recovering from COVID-19, NAC has shown potential benefits. A randomized clinical trial demonstrated that NAC supplementation in children with moderate COVID-19 improved oxygen saturation levels and reduced hospital stay durations. Additionally, NAC's antioxidant and anti-inflammatory properties may help alleviate neurological symptoms such as brain fog, which are common in Long COVID. Preliminary findings suggest that combining NAC with other treatments could enhance cognitive functioning in Long COVID patients. (9)

Important:

While NAC is generally considered safe for children, it's essential to consult a healthcare provider before initiating supplementation. Potential side effects include gastrointestinal discomfort, and there may be interactions with other medications. NAC should be used cautiously in children with asthma or bleeding disorders, as it may exacerbate these conditions. Monitoring by a healthcare professional ensures appropriate dosing and minimizes risks.

Dosage Guidelines:

There are no official pediatric dosing guidelines for NAC; however, some practitioners recommend the following:

- **Young children:** Up to 300 mg twice daily

- **Teenagers:** Up to 600 mg twice daily

Sulfate

Why It's Helpful

Sulfate is an essential nutrient for many body processes. It plays a key role in mitochondrial energy production, the sulfation detoxification pathway in the liver, and the formation of connective tissues, cartilage, and the gut lining. For children with Long COVID, sulfate can be especially important because prolonged illness, high inflammation, and disrupted gut function may reduce the body's ability to recycle or generate enough sulfate. Adequate sulfate helps support immune regulation, brain health, and cellular energy, which are often disrupted in post-viral recovery.

Important

Not all sulfate sources are equally suitable for children, especially those with digestive sensitivities. Some oral sulfate salts (such as magnesium sulfate/Epsom salts) act as strong laxatives and may worsen diarrhea, which is already a problem for many Long COVID patients. Instead, gentler sources are preferred, such as:

- Zinc sulfate (oral or topical lotion/cream): Provides both zinc (immune and gut healing benefits) and sulfate in a well-tolerated form. Topical zinc sulfate lotion may be particularly helpful for children with sensitive digestion.

- Epsom salt (magnesium sulfate) baths: Transdermal absorption provides sulfate without the laxative effect of oral use. These baths can also help relax muscles and promote better sleep.
- Dietary sources: Cruciferous vegetables (broccoli, cauliflower, Brussels sprouts), onions, and garlic naturally contain sulfur compounds that the body can convert to sulfate.
- Caution: Oral magnesium sulfate should be avoided in children with diarrhea, dehydration, or kidney disease. Zinc supplementation beyond recommended limits may interfere with copper absorption, so long-term use should be monitored by a clinician.
- Because sulfate works alongside magnesium and thiamine, many clinicians recommend using them together to support energy recovery and mitochondrial function in children with Long COVID.

Dosing Guidelines

- Zinc sulfate (oral): Typical pediatric dosing is 1–2 mg/kg/day of elemental zinc (not the total salt), up to 20 mg/day for young children and up to 40 mg/day in adolescents, unless otherwise directed by a physician.
- Zinc sulfate (topical lotion): Safe when applied once daily to intact skin; dosing is less precise but useful in children who cannot tolerate oral zinc.
- Epsom salt (magnesium sulfate) baths: ½ to 1 cup of Epsom salt in a warm bath, 2–3 times per week, is a common regimen for children. Duration should be about 10–20 minutes, supervised.

- Dietary sulfate: Encourage regular intake of sulfur-rich foods such as broccoli, kale, onions, and garlic as a natural, steady source of sulfate.

Thiamine

Why It's Helpful:

Thiamine, also known as vitamin B1, is an essential nutrient that helps cells produce energy(10). It is found naturally in a variety of foods, including pork (lean cuts or organ meats), whole grains, legumes, sunflower seeds, flax seeds, pistachios, asparagus, spinach, and kale, to name a few. Brewer's and nutritional yeast gets a special mention as it is extremely high in thiamine(11).

Thiamine is particularly important for the nervous system, heart, and muscles, acting like a spark plug for the body's cellular "batteries." Without enough thiamine, children can develop symptoms similar to beriberi, a condition historically associated with severe deficiency(12).

Wet beriberi affects the heart and blood vessels, causing swelling (edema), rapid heart rate, difficulty breathing, and, in severe cases, heart failure because the heart doesn't have enough energy to pump effectively (12,13).

Dry beriberi primarily affects the nervous system, leading to numbness, tingling, pain, weakness, or difficulty walking(12,13).

In pediatric Long COVID, some children experience fatigue, palpitations, dizziness, exercise intolerance, or brain fog. These symptoms may closely resemble POTS, which may cause confusion(14). Research suggests that thiamine deficiency may contribute to these symptoms, especially when prolonged illness increases the body's energy demand or when absorption and intake are reduced(15,16).

Thiamine may be closely connected to Long COVID because of its essential role in energy production, nerve function, and immune health(16,17). When thiamine levels are low, children can feel unusually tired, weak, or mentally foggy, which mirrors the common fatigue and brain fog reported after COVID-19(14,17). Severe infections often trigger high levels of inflammation, which can quickly deplete thiamine stores, leaving some children deficient even after recovery(16).

Since thiamine is a cofactor in the citric acid cycle, a key pathway that generates cellular energy (ATP), deficiency can disrupt metabolism and further worsen fatigue(10,16). Thiamine also supports a healthy immune response, so inadequate levels may reduce antibody production or immune defense(17). Encouragingly, small studies have found that thiamine supplementation may ease lingering post-COVID symptoms such as fatigue, muscle pain, and sleep disturbances, highlighting its potential role in recovery(18).

Important:

Thiamine works best when combined with magnesium and sulfate.

- Magnesium is required to convert thiamine into its active form, thiamine pyrophosphate. Without magnesium, even high doses of thiamine may be less effective(19).
- If magnesium is not supplemented, the body may remove the magnesium from the blood or the bones, resulting in weakened bones and other deficiencies(19).

- Sulfate supports energy pathways in the mitochondria and helps the body use thiamine efficiently.

Many clinicians recommend supplementing all three together—thiamine, magnesium, and sulfate—for optimal benefit in children recovering from Long COVID(18).

Dosing Guidelines

Oral supplementation (weight- and age-based):

Age Group	Typical Oral Dose
Infants 0–6 months	0.2–0.3 mg/kg/day
Children 7 months–3 years	0.5–1 mg/kg/day
Children 4–10 years	1–1.5 mg/kg/day
Adolescents 11+ years	25–50 mg/day (higher doses 100–200 mg/day under supervision)

IV Thiamine (for severe deficiency):

Indicated if the child has cardiac symptoms (rapid heartbeat, edema, shortness of breath) or cannot tolerate oral intake(12,13).

If a child has symptoms (encephalopathy, ataxia, ophthalmoplegia, cardiomyopathy, lactic acidosis, unexplained irritability/neuropathy): IV thiamine is indicated immediately, without waiting for level confirmation.

If a child is high-risk but asymptomatic (refeeding, prolonged TPN without vitamins, severe malnutrition, hyperemesis, oncology patient, chronic GI disease), many guidelines recommend empiric IV thiamine even if a level isn't yet available(20).

If a level comes back low but the child is clinically stable and can tolerate enteral/oral therapy, oral supplementation is often sufficient.

Typical hospital dosing:

- Infants: 10–25 mg IV daily
- Older children: 25–100 mg IV daily

Continue until symptoms improve and oral intake is possible. IV administration should always be done under medical supervision, with careful monitoring of heart and electrolytes.

Ivermectin Use (Off-label and Under Clinical Supervision Only)

Why it's helpful:

Ivermectin may play a role in modulating the immune response and reducing inflammation. Ivermectin has been proposed as a potential treatment for long COVID due to several theoretical mechanisms, although robust clinical evidence is still limited and often debated. Here's how it may help, according to early hypotheses and small studies:

1. **Antiviral Action**: Ivermectin has demonstrated antiviral activity *in vitro* against a range of viruses (21), including

SARS-CoV-2. Some researchers speculate that residual viral proteins may persist in long COVID patients, and ivermectin could help reduce this viral load.

2. **Anti-inflammatory Effects**: Chronic inflammation is thought to play a role in long COVID. Research indicates that ivermectin may exert anti-inflammatory effects by inhibiting the production of pro-inflammatory cytokines such as interleukin-6 (IL-6) and tumor necrosis factor-alpha (TNF-α) (22). In a study by Zhang et al. (2008), ivermectin significantly decreased the production of TNF-α, IL-1β, and IL-6 in both in vivo and in vitro models. The study demonstrated that ivermectin suppressed lipopolysaccharide (LPS)-induced nuclear factor-kappa B (NF-κB) translocation, a key pathway in the inflammatory response, thereby reducing cytokine production. These findings suggest that ivermectin may help modulate an overactive immune response, which is thought to play a role in long COVID.

3. **Immunomodulation**: Research suggests that ivermectin may modulate immune function by interacting with Toll-like receptor (TLR) pathways, which are crucial in the body's innate immune response. Specifically, ivermectin has been shown to inhibit the activation of TLR4, a receptor that, when stimulated, can lead to the production of pro-inflammatory cytokines such as IL-6 and TNF-α. By suppressing TLR4 activation, ivermectin may help reduce excessive inflammatory responses. For instance, a study demonstrated that ivermectin treatment led to decreased expression of TLR4 in a rat model of vasculitis, suggesting its potential to modulate immune signaling pathways associated with inflammation(23). Additionally, ivermectin's influence

on TLR pathways may contribute to rebalancing immune function disrupted in conditions like long COVID. By dampening overactive immune responses and promoting a more regulated cytokine production, ivermectin could theoretically aid in restoring normal immune signaling.

4. **Anticoagulant and Microclot Reduction**: Emerging research suggests that ivermectin may influence blood clotting pathways, potentially impacting the formation of microclots associated with long COVID. A computational study by Boschi et al. (2023) utilized molecular docking and dynamics simulations to explore ivermectin's interaction with fibrinogen, a key protein in clot formation. The study found that ivermectin could bind to multiple sites on the fibrinogen molecule, particularly in regions critical for its interaction with the SARS-CoV-2 spike protein. By potentially interfering with this binding, ivermectin may reduce the formation of abnormal fibrin clots that are resistant to degradation, which have been implicated in the pathology of long COVID. The authors concluded that these findings warrant further in vitro and in vivo studies to validate ivermectin's role in modulating thrombo-inflammatory processes associated with long COVID (24).

5. **Neurological Protection**: Research indicates that ivermectin may modulate neurotransmission and reduce neuroinflammation, which could be relevant for addressing neurological symptoms associated with long COVID, such as brain fog. One study demonstrated that ivermectin treatment in a murine model of cerebral toxoplasmosis significantly increased the expression of γ-aminobutyric acid (GABA) in brain tissue and

improved cerebral histopathology (25). This suggests that ivermectin may influence GABAergic neurotransmission, potentially contributing to neuroprotective effects.

While these findings are promising, it's important to note that they are based on preclinical models. Further research is necessary to confirm these effects in humans and to explore the potential role of ivermectin in managing neurological symptoms of long COVID.

Important:

- Any use of ivermectin in pediatric cases must be supervised by a qualified healthcare provider and comply with local regulations and clinical best practices.
- Initiate only under strict medical supervision and with careful monitoring. Ivermectin dosage is very specific and based on body weight.
- Discontinue or adjust if no improvement is observed within a few weeks. Note that some patients will report no improvement, but will report a worsening of symptoms if Ivermectin is discontinued. This means that the Ivermectin most likely *was* helping and should be continued.
- Some children may show delayed responses or sensitivity to dose changes.
- Due to the possible drug interaction between quercetin and ivermectin, these drugs should not be taken simultaneously (i.e., should be staggered morning and night).
- Long-term use decisions should weigh benefits vs. potential risks and side effects. It is important to note

that current scientific evidence does not support the use of ivermectin for treating pediatric long COVID. Major health organizations, including the FDA and the Infectious Diseases Society of America (IDSA), advise against using ivermectin for COVID-19 treatment outside of clinical trials due to insufficient evidence of its efficacy and potential risks.

Low-Dose Naltrexone (LDN)

Why it's helpful:

Low-dose naltrexone (LDN) is being explored as a potential treatment for long COVID due to its immunomodulatory and anti-inflammatory properties. Studies have reported that LDN may alleviate symptoms such as fatigue, pain, cognitive dysfunction, and sleep disturbances in long COVID patients. For instance, a study involving 52 patients treated with LDN observed improvements in activities of daily living, energy levels, pain, concentration, and sleep disturbances. Another study reported that patients taking LDN experienced significant improvements in fatigue and pain compared to those receiving physical therapy alone. These findings suggest that LDN may help rebalance immune function and reduce neuroinflammation, potentially addressing some of the underlying mechanisms of long COVID (26).

Important:

- Initiate only under medical supervision and with careful monitoring following clinical best practices.
- Onset of effects can take 2–3 months. Monitor closely for side effects and **ensure no concurrent opioid use.**

- Always compounded: LDN must be prepared by a compounding pharmacy in liquid or capsule form to achieve accurate low doses.
- Best taken at night: It may support immune function during sleep, but some children tolerate it better in the morning.

General Pediatric LDN Dosing Guidelines:

Typical Starting Dose (Weight-Based): 0.025 to 0.05 mg/kg/day, usually given at bedtime. For example:

Starting dose:

- A 20 kg (44 lb) child might start at **0.5 to 1 mg nightly**.
- A 30 kg (66 lb) child might start at **0.75 to 1.5 mg nightly**.
- **Titration:** Increase slowly every 1–2 weeks, by 0.25–0.5 mg, based on: Symptom improvement and side effects (e.g., vivid dreams, irritability)
- Some children may respond well to doses as low as 0.5 mg.
- The maximum pediatric dose usually should not exceed 3 mg/day.

Usual Maintenance Range:

- **1 to 3 mg nightly**, depending on age, weight, and clinical response.

Hyperbaric Oxygen Therapy

Hyperbaric oxygen therapy (HBOT) is emerging as a potential treatment for pediatric Long COVID, particularly for addressing symptoms like fatigue, cognitive dysfunction, and persistent inflammation. HBOT involves breathing 100% oxygen in a pressurized environment, which significantly increases oxygen delivery to tissues, promoting healing and reducing inflammatory processes. A 2022 randomized controlled trial by Zilberman-Itskovich et al. demonstrated that HBOT significantly improved cognitive function, energy levels, and psychiatric symptoms in adults suffering from post-COVID-19 conditions (27). While research in pediatric populations is still limited, early case reports and extrapolations from studies in conditions like traumatic brain injury suggest that children may experience similar neurocognitive and physical benefits (Harch, *Medical Gas Research*, 2020). Given the pressing need for effective treatments for pediatric Long COVID, HBOT represents a promising option that warrants further clinical study.

Rezzimax

The Rezzimax® is a simple handheld device that vibrates in a very specific way, using different wavelengths resembling the vibrations that cats produce when they purr. We use it in our program in various ways and find it extremely effective. The Rezzimax® device may offer a valuable tool for supporting children recovering from Long COVID, especially for managing symptoms like headaches, muscle tension, and autonomic nervous system dysfunction (such as fatigue, dizziness, and anxiety). The device uses targeted vibration, resonance, and gentle pressure to stimulate the vagus nerve and relax tight muscles in the face, neck, and upper body. In pediatric Long COVID, where persistent autonomic imbalance and chronic pain are often reported, gentle vagus nerve stimulation may help regulate stress responses, improve circulation, and reduce inflammation. While formal studies specifically on Rezzimax use in pediatric Long COVID are not yet available, research on vagus nerve stimulation in children with conditions like migraines and dysautonomia suggests potential benefits (28). Given its non-invasive nature and ease of use, Rezzimax therapy may serve as a supportive adjunct to broader rehabilitation programs aimed at restoring function and improving quality of life in young Long COVID patients.

Cereset

Cereset is a non-invasive, non-pharmaceutical neurotechnology designed to help the brain achieve greater balance and resilience, which may offer benefits for children suffering from long COVID symptoms such as brain fog, sleep disturbances, anxiety, and fatigue. Cereset uses BrainEcho® technology, translating real-time brainwave patterns into auditory tones that are fed back to the individual. This gentle biofeedback may help the brain self-correct imbalances and promote improved autonomic regulation.

In a randomized, controlled study, Cereset was shown to significantly improve sleep quality and autonomic function in adults with insomnia, as measured by improvements in heart rate variability and Pittsburgh Sleep Quality Index scores (29). Although pediatric-specific studies are still emerging, early case reports suggest similar potential for improving cognitive and emotional symptoms in children by optimizing brain rhythm balance. Given that long COVID often involves autonomic dysregulation and disrupted sleep in children, Cereset may represent a promising supportive therapy. Families should consult with a knowledgeable healthcare provider before starting Cereset to ensure it fits into an individualized treatment plan.

Exercise With Oxygen Therapy (EWOT)

EWOT offers an exciting, evidence-informed option to support recovery in children with Long COVID. It is also a therapy that we include as part of our program. EWOT combines physical exercise with high-flow oxygen, significantly improving oxygen delivery to tissues. This can help boost energy levels, reduce inflammation, and restore stamina — critical goals for young patients facing persistent symptoms. Research has shown that oxygen-supplemented exercise improves cardiovascular function and reduces fatigue in individuals with chronic health conditions (30).

We also know that Long COVID often disrupts the body's ability to use oxygen efficiently (31), making targeted therapies like EWOT especially relevant. While more pediatric-specific studies are needed, EWOT is a safe, proactive, and promising addition to a comprehensive rehabilitation program. It empowers children to rebuild strength at their own pace while offering families hope for a smoother, faster recovery.

Soliman Auricular Allergy Treatment (SAAT)

Soliman Auricular Allergy Treatment (SAAT) is a specialized form of ear acupuncture that uses a single, semi-permanent needle placed at a precise point to modulate the immune response. Originally designed to address severe allergies, SAAT has shown promising results in conditions involving immune system dysregulation and inflammation — two key components believed to underlie pediatric long COVID. By influencing the autonomic nervous system and reducing inflammatory markers, SAAT may help children struggling with persistent symptoms like fatigue, brain fog, digestive problems, and respiratory issues.

Auricular acupuncture has been found in clinical studies to improve vagal tone, reduce inflammatory cytokines, and rebalance autonomic function (32). Although formal studies on SAAT specifically for long COVID are still limited, case series and clinical reports suggest it can provide meaningful symptom relief in complex, immune-mediated conditions. Because SAAT typically requires only one needle placement per treatment trigger and carries minimal risk when performed by a trained practitioner, it is an efficient, targeted option for pediatric patients needing gentle yet powerful immune support.

How to Implement:

Being in charge of a loved one's care can be intimidating. Below, I have planned out a sample care plan, stretched over an entire year. While our program lasts approximately 14 weeks only, it is important to know that unless you have the tools to handle unpleasant side effects from treatments, such as detoxification side effects, it is best to take the slow and steady route. Stick to it and be patient. My dad always says, "nervous cats make bad jumps". Be methodical and keep notes. Above all, be patient and believe that, innately, your child's body was designed to heal. Sometimes, it just needs some help from the outside.

Here's a carefully phased 1-year integrative treatment plan for pediatric Long COVID using the therapies, medications, supplements, and vitamins listed above. This approach balances safety, synergy, and clinical impact — avoiding overwhelming your child's body by staggering introductions and prioritizing foundational support first.

Treatment Principles:

- Start low, go slow. Introduce no more than 1–2 new interventions every 2 weeks.

- Monitor your child's response and adjust based on symptoms, labs, or side effects.

- Emphasize foundational care first, then move to mitochondrial, neurological, and immune-specific therapies.

- Every child is different. Work with your child's healthcare professional and monitor their progress as indicated below (for example, by having their labs checked).

SAMPLE YEARLONG PEDIATRIC LONG COVID PLAN (Divided by Quarter)

Month 1–3: Foundation & Gut Reset

Goal: Stabilize gut, improve absorption, reduce inflammation

- **Simple Spectrum**
(daily; start with 1/8th of a scoop and increase slowly as tolerated)

- **Probiotics + Gut Support**
(daily; multi-strain pediatric-specific)

- **IGG Food Sensitivity Treatment**
(Elimination diet based on testing OR trial gluten/dairy reduction)

- **Magnesium**
(Start 100–200 mg magnesium glycinate at bedtime)

- **Test for thiamine deficiency and supplement if appropriate** (See page 106)

- **Manganese**
  (Start with 0.5mg and work up to 2mg)

- **Vitamins D3 + K2**
  (Daily: D3 ~1000–2000 IU with K2)

- **Methylated B Vitamins**
  (Low-dose B12 and methylfolate 3x/week to start; ramp to daily)

- **Minerals**
  (Zinc, selenium, trace mineral mix OR targeted based on labs)

- **Cereset treatment©** (If available in your area, as prescribed by practitioner after completing baseline scan)

Month 4–6: Mitochondrial & Cognitive Support

Goal: Enhance energy, reduce oxidative stress, address brain fog

- **NAC**
  (Begin 300–600 mg/day, titrate slowly)

- **Melatonin**
  (0.5–3 mg at bedtime if sleep issues persist; also antioxidant benefits)

- **Blue-Green Algae**
  (Low-dose, nutrient support if tolerable; optional if diet is already nutrient-dense)

- **EWOT (Exercise With Oxygen Therapy)**
  (2–3x/week, short sessions under guidance; build tolerance gradually)

- **Rezzimax©** for vagus nerve stimulation.

Month 7–9: Immune Modulation & Advanced Therapies

Goal: Regulate overactive immune system, address microclotting & lingering symptoms

- **Low Dose Naltrexone (LDN)**
  (Start 0.5 mg, titrate up to 1.5–3 mg nightly)

- **SAAT Acupuncture**
  (Weekly or bi-weekly sessions, depending on response)

- **Nattokinase**
  (Begin low-dose every other day; avoid if bleeding disorders)

- **Hyperbaric Oxygen Therapy (HBOT)**
  (1–2x/week, 20–40 sessions depending on response and tolerance)

- **Gentle physical therapy (such as pool therapy)**
  If your child can tolerate it. Start slowly and build up.

Month 10–12: Antiviral & Regenerative Phase

Goal: Tackle residual inflammation, promote cellular repair

- **Ivermectin (if clinically indicated)**
  (Use cautiously, only under a knowledgeable provider's care)

- **BPC-157 (oral or topical)**
  (Consider for persistent gut, nerve, or muscle repair; 2–4 week trial)
  fatigue or cognition)

Ongoing Throughout the Year

- **Recheck labs every 3–6 months**: Vitamins D/B12, homocysteine, zinc, CRP, CBC, thyroid, etc.

- **Track symptom response** with a weekly log (energy, mood, sleep, pain, cognition).

- **Work with a functional or integrative pediatric provider** for dosing and interactions.

Be patient — healing is not linear. It's natural to want fast results, but recovery often comes in slow, subtle waves. At first, you may not even notice the progress. Improvements might feel small or inconsistent, but over time, they build. Study the patterns. Look for the quiet wins. Even on the hard days — when it feels like nothing is working — remember: every positive choice you make supports your child's healing. Nutrients, therapies, rest, love — they all add up, even if the effects aren't immediate.

There will be setbacks. That's normal. But don't let them steal your hope. Perseverance matters more than perfection. What you're doing takes courage. And while you can't control every outcome, you *can* keep showing up with intention. Change happens when we do things differently. Keep going. You are planting seeds that will grow in time. You have very little to lose and everything to gain.

Chapter 9:
Patient stories

"Although the world is full of suffering, it is also full of the overcoming of it."

Helen Keller

"The human spirit is stronger than anything that can happen to it."

C.C. Scott

Dylan's Long Covid Story

The perfect storm led to my son losing his life for nearly three years. Our son was an 11-year-old boy who loved playing soccer and basketball, had lots of friends, straight A's in school, and, except for seasonal allergies, was completely healthy. In January of 2022, that all changed when I caught Covid for the first time, five days later, so did my son. We both had mild symptoms for about two weeks. He suffered from body aches, congestion, cough, headache, and a low-grade fever. After two weeks, he was completely fine and returned to school, caught up on all of his missed work, and even finished out the basketball season.

On February 17, 2022, just four days after his 12th birthday, Long COVID symptoms started (we didn't know that at the time) with congestion, a runny nose, and a horrible cough. He missed a few days of school, and when he wasn't showing any signs of getting better, I took him to the doctor for the first time on 2/22/22. That was the first of many trips over the next few months. Doctors at that time were not familiar with Long Covid, and he was diagnosed with a sinus infection, walking pneumonia, and a habit cough. After many rounds of blood tests that all came back clear, my son's PCP started sending us

"

to specialists. From February to June, my son saw an infectious disease doctor, a cardiologist, a pulmonary doctor, had three ER visits, and a functional medicine doctor. Still no answers to why our son was getting more ill every day.

Finally, we thought there was hope when a Long Covid clinic called us. We had been on the waiting list for months, hoping for a call. On June 16, 2022, we drove two hours to the clinic and saw a team of about eight doctors, ranging from a nutritionist to a neurologist. By the time we made it to the clinic, our son had severe nerve pain, could no longer walk, migraines, brain fog, cough, fatigue, and was very weak. He also could no longer attend school. We were so desperate to find some type of help for our son. After a full eight hours at the Long Covid clinic, we left there with a prescription of Gabapentin and at-home PT. They also recommended putting him on their waiting list for an inpatient program where he would have stayed at the hospital for 6-8 weeks alone. He would not have been able to see us, and we could only talk to him for 20 minutes a day on the phone. They said this was to focus completely on therapy and getting him well. We said absolutely NOT! Our son couldn't walk and couldn't take care of himself. We were not going to leave him with complete strangers who still couldn't tell me what our son was suffering from. Needless to say, we were looked down upon for not agreeing to this program.

By July of 2022, the Long Covid team of doctors was just increasing his Gabapentin (which was not helping). He also continued with PT at home. Our son was bedridden and had developed slurred speech from the side effects of the high dose of medication. I was in constant contact with his doctors, and they just kept pushing the inpatient program. By the end of

July, one of the Long Covid doctors (a neurologist) referred Dylan to an inpatient rehabilitation program at another hospital that allowed a parent to stay with their child. We agreed to this program, and on August 9th, 2022, we headed to the rehabilitation center.

We had such high hopes, and so did Dylan. I was the one staying with Dylan at the rehabilitation center. When we arrived, our son was in a wheelchair because of how weak he had become and was unable to walk. His days were filled with PT, OT, speech, and CBT. Within 24 hours, Dylan could no longer hold his body upright, sit up, or control any movement. We arrived on a Tuesday evening, and by Friday morning, after seeing an OT therapist for 10 minutes, he was diagnosed with FND (functional neurological disorder). This was a therapist who had taken a weekend workshop on FND. She then spoke to the head doctor, and he agreed that it was the final diagnosis. Needless to say, I did not agree!

Long story short, we were at the rehabilitation center for four weeks. Within that time, Dylan had lost the ability to move, speak, and swallow. It was two weeks of not being able to swallow, the doctor would not allow a feeding tube because he was treating it as a behavior issue. I even had to fight with them to keep his food in his room for me to try feeding him. Our hopes were to take home our son feeling better, but instead, our son was basically a vegetable. We returned home on September 8th, 2022.

Dylan's body was starting to shut down! Not long after returning home, Dylan had to stay in a children's hospital for 10 days to get an NG feeding tube because he still couldn't eat or drink. While at the children's hospital, he started having short spells that looked like seizures. Later, to find out the short spells were non-epileptic seizures caused by pain and trauma, not only from Long Covid but from the abuse he endured at the rehabilitation children's hospital. The only positives were that our son was finally getting the nutrition he needed, and he began to speak to my husband and me. The joy of hearing his voice after almost two months was unbelievable.

After the non-epileptic seizures began, Dylan began to isolate himself from all family and friends except for his father and me. His psychologist said he was doing that because he didn't want others to see what he had become after getting sick, it was a form of protecting himself.

Each day, our son was just getting worse, and there was no one who knew how to help him. All the doctors wanted to do was give him antidepressants. By this point, I had stopped teaching to give full-time care to our son. All I did besides taking care of my son was research and read! I had to find someone who could help him. But that never happened!

It was May of 2023, our 13-year-old son was completely bedridden, had a feeding tube, full body nerve pain, blurred and double vision, ringing in his ears, migraines, had 50-100 non-epileptic seizures a day, dissociated, had violent rages, couldn't feel the urge to urinate, anxiety, depression, and PTSD from all of the pain and trauma. As Dylan said before, we were just surviving, not living! I just knew that something bad was going to happen to either Dylan or me because of all of his non-epileptic seizures, violent rages, and dissociation.

Daily, I had to hold him down from attacking me and destroying the room. While he dissociated, he would black out. I suffered from two concussions, several black eyes from objects being thrown, and we both had scratches and bruises. This life we were living was hell, and I couldn't save him, no matter how hard I tried. The look in my son's eyes after coming out of a non-epileptic seizure and after dissociating was a look of horror. He was so scared and ashamed of what he had done, but couldn't control or stop the spells.

Throughout all of his illness, I was in weekly contact with his psychologist, who guided me through all of Dylan's emotional trauma. Remember, as I stated above, Dylan's anxiety and PTSD prevented him from seeing or talking to anyone other than his father and me. Every week, Dylan's wonderful psychologist talked and explained to me what was happening to our son. Honestly, at times, I don't think I would have survived if it hadn't been for his knowledge, kindness, and compassion for Dylan and our family. I also met every three months with his GI doctor, psychiatrist, and PCP for check-ins.

Finally, after a year and a half, I had convinced Dylan's psychiatrist (I sent him all of the research I had found on LDN) to prescribe him Low Dose Naltrexone (LDN). I had read many articles and researched how LDN was helping LC patients with pain, anxiety, PTSD, and dissociation. The last thing I wanted to do was to try another medication because of how Dylan had responded to all of the others, but we had no other choice. He started LDN at a very low dose, .50 mg, and every two weeks I increased it by .25 mg with the hope of it helping in some way. Within 4 weeks, Dylan went from having 50-100 non-epileptic seizures a day to only having one when he was picked up or carried to bed or the bathroom due to the pain. Although our son was still so ill, with the non-epileptic seizures and dissociation stopping, we were able to breathe a little. We were hoping for more improvements, but sadly, that didn't happen.

When the new school year of 2023 started, Dylan had missed all of 7th grade and was now missing the start of his 8th-grade year. He missed his friends, playing sports, reading, playing games, field trips, school dances, and just laughing and being a kid. It broke our hearts as parents to see our sweet little boy missing out on all of these special moments that he could never get back. He missed the last few years of his precious childhood. Our days were spent in one room upstairs in our home. Because of Dylan's anxiety and PTSD, he had not left the house since November 2022. He wouldn't even go downstairs. Daily, we felt like we were losing our son and felt helpless. No one could help heal our son because Long Covid was such a new diagnosis.

Since I had stayed home for Dylan's full-time care for the school year 2022-23, my husband and I decided that I needed to return part-time to teaching in 2023. We were lucky that my husband was able to work from home two days a week. We were blessed that the school where I worked and Dylan attended treated us like family. They had me come two days a week to be the STREAM teacher for grades 1-5. This allowed Dylan to depend on someone else besides me, and helped Dylan and his father get closer again. I also needed socialization!

In February of 2024, I caught Covid for the second time and, of course, gave it to Dylan. With every illness, from a cold to the flu, Dylan's symptoms worsened. I was terrified of what getting Covid again would do to our sweet boy, and I was right to be terrified. His symptoms worsened which I couldn't even imagine could have been possible. He was completely bedridden, could not move at all, and developed severe nausea, vomiting, and stomach pain. He couldn't even focus on watching TV, which was even too painful for him. We were totally lost at this point and had no clue how to help our son. COVID wasn't going anywhere, it was here to stay. I kept asking my husband how he would live and survive like this.

Finally, on March 5th of 2024, I received a text from my long-term sub (yes, my school had been holding my position for two years), not a doctor, not from researching, my long-term sub gave us the information we needed. God had a plan, and it was starting! She told me of a clinic in Fayetteville, Arkansas, that was starting to help Long Covid patients. Her sister had known someone with some of the same symptoms as Dylan, who had just graduated from the clinic completely in remission. But the only problem was that health insurance wouldn't pay for it. At that point, my heart sank, and I thought how could we even think about paying for this. Even with all of my hesitation, my husband and I said we had to try, we had to save our son's life.

The next day, I filled out the online form, and by that afternoon, someone had contacted me. I'm not going to lie, I actually avoided the call because I thought this had to be too good to be true, and I didn't want to disappoint our son again or give him false hope. Finally, the clinic reached my husband, and he was the first to talk to them. He was very excited when he was telling me about what they could do to help Dylan get his life back. My husband said you have to talk to them tomorrow. The next day, I spoke to the most amazing lady, she was so kind, soft spoken, she listened, and she believed me. She said that they could help and told me about several Long COVID cases they had helped since 2023. She also put me in contact with another Spero mom already at the clinic on week 8 with her son, who was the same age as Dylan, got sick at the same time, and had most of the same symptoms as Dylan. When we talked, we cried, we laughed, and we shared our stories. I thought to myself that if the clinic is anything like the young lady I spoke to, it would be amazing. We finally had hope! For almost three years, we had been searching for help to heal our son with no answers. For the next 12 weeks, the Spero mom and I kept in touch. She told me weekly about her son's wins and challenges, about what the therapies would cost per week, and described how she felt as a mother seeing her son go through this journey. She was a true angel to me!

After multiple conversations and even a Zoom call with Dr. K, the lead doctor, we decided to schedule a start date for Dylan, June 26, 2024. We had three months to raise enough money for the treatment and our relocation to Arkansas. Between my husband and me, we contacted our local newspaper, radio, and TV stations. We brought awareness to Long Covid, our son's story, and the fact that health insurance would not cover the medical care our son needed to get well. But what feared us most was how in the world we would tell Dylan what our plan was. How would we tell him, with his anxiety, depression, and PTSD, that we were taking him to another medical facility to try to heal him, that we were leaving our home he hadn't left in 18 months, that we were staying in Arkansas for who knows how long. We knew that he would refuse to go, and he would be mad at us for planning this and even thinking the clinic could help. Needless to say, my anxiety was bad, but my husband just had the attitude that we were going to do this and that it would be ok!

After speaking to Dylan's psychologist, he agreed that if we told him right away and gave him three months to worry and fear the trip, it would not be healthy for Dylan. We decided to tell him a week before leaving for Arkansas. But Dylan's psychologist did say that we needed to get him out of the house for a short weekend trip before our journey to Arkansas. My husband and I had discussed ways of traveling to Arkansas and where to stay while we relocated. Dylan was not able to sit up in a car and definitely couldn't fly in a plane, so we decided to drive an RV to Arkansas. Dylan would be able to lay in the bed for the trip, and we would also be able to bring our three dogs on the journey. Honestly, staying in an RV saved us on living expenses as well.

Dylan's first trip out of the house in 18 months was challenging to say the least! The only thing leading up to our weekend getaway, we told Dylan, was that we had purchased an RV for camping. As a family, we always loved camping, so he was actually happy! Two days before leaving in May of 2024 for our getaway, we told Dylan that we were going to Ocean City camping in our new RV. He screamed NOOOOOO and that he wasn't going and that we couldn't make him. We knew this was the reaction that he would have, and we knew after telling him the details of our trip that we just needed to leave him alone to process what was happening.

The plan was to leave on Tuesday, May 21, 2024, and only stay until Thursday. On the day we were leaving, Dylan kept having non-epileptic seizures and dissociating; he was so terrified. His therapist said to talk to Dylan prior to making a plan and doing anything that would make him more comfortable/safe when leaving the house for the first time. Dylan said that because he hadn't been downstairs in a long time, it brought back bad memories—specifically from when he returned from the children's hospital after almost dying. He said that he wanted to be blindfolded before being carried downstairs. The whole time my husband was carrying him to the RV, he was yelling no, and dissociating/blacking out.

Finally, we were on our way, and it was a rough start, but finally Dylan settled down, and after the hour drive to Ocean City with the dogs in his lap, I think I saw a smile. We were only supposed to stay for two nights, but Dylan first said let's stay until Friday so we did, then he said let's stay until Monday so we did! Dylan stayed in the RV and stayed in bed, but just getting out of the house and seeing new things, people, smells, and sounds out of his window was so amazing for him. He had overcome a huge fear of leaving the bedroom and the house he had been in for 18 months. We knew we were on the right track.

Now the countdown was on, we had less than one month before leaving for Arkansas. Three days before leaving, we told Dylan we had to talk to him. He knew we had been planning something with buying the RV. I had been telling him success stories of patients recovering from Long Covid, and by going camping, he knew something was up. His reaction was not as strong as his first reaction when we told him we were going camping. He was still angry and didn't want to hear much about our plan because he didn't believe anything would work. He said, "It has worked for others, but that doesn't mean it will heal me." He then asked, "Please leave me alone so I can process this." In the final days, I had to pack Dylan's belongings and he would actually tell me things to pack. June 19th finally arrived and we proceeded in the same way as we did when we went camping. Dylan wanted us to blindfold him and my husband had to carry him to the RV. He laid in the bed with the three dogs as we began our journey to heal our son.

Needless to say, our journey in the RV with a sick child and three dogs, in the summer heat, was a challenge but we did it. We arrived in Fayetteville, Arkansas June 25 and Dylan started at The Spero Clinic on June 26, 2024. The night we arrived Dylan wanted me to cut his hair that hadn't been cut in over two years (it was long). I also had been giving him sponge baths for the last two years because of his nerve pain and not being able to hold himself up. That night he wanted me to really clean him for the next day, he endured the pain. We even picked out an outfit for the next day! We were ready but I was still so scared of how things were going to go. Was Dylan too sick for them to heal, how was he going to stay in a wheelchair all day and follow a schedule when he could barely lay in bed, how would he wear clothes when his nerve pain was so severe, how would we feed him with his feeding tube during therapies, and how would he handle seeing and hearing people when he hadn't interacted with people in over 18 months? The morning of the 26th arrived and there was a huge thunderstorm that morning which just added to our obstacles. That morning we did our normal routines and I got him dressed. My husband started the handicap van and then came in to pick up Dylan to carry him to the van. I was expecting him to have a non-epileptic seizure, dissociate/blackout, and yell like he had each time we put him in the RV for our trips but he didn't. He just closed his eyes and let my husband, his dad carry him to his wheelchair in the van. He was willing to go and that in itself was a huge success! We had finally made it to The Spero Clinic and were so hopeful!

8:30 am on June 26, 2024, Dylan started his day at the clinic. When we entered the door, the front desk staff was so welcoming and had smiles on their faces. Then we went to intake with an amazing and caring woman who made us all feel so welcome. At one point, Dylan looked at me, and I knew that meant he needed a break. Remember, he wouldn't talk to anyone else but me and his dad. His dad took him to the bathroom, and he was actually fine, he just needed to go to the bathroom. We were so amazed at how well he was handling all of this. His first day was a full day of therapies and meetings about what to expect. We met his amazing doctor and all of his therapists, and they were all extremely caring and kind. Spero was unlike any place we had ever been to before. By the end of the first day, Dylan had cooperated with all the therapists and was willing to try all that was asked of him. We were so happy and so exhausted! After the first week, Dylan dropped a bomb on us. He stated that he didn't want to live anymore with this pain, and he had felt this way for a long time. We talked for hours as a family, and I also talked to his therapist. He said that Dylan had been through so much, and now this journey at the clinic has probably overwhelmed him. Believe me, we took his statement seriously and watched him carefully. We also knew that at some point in his therapies, he would get help for his PTSD. As the weeks continued, we just saw more small improvements and smiles.

The first six weeks, we saw mental and emotional breakthroughs. Dylan started talking to his NMR therapist within the first week and then to his doctors the second week. He was texting his friends, and as a family we were able to go to the grocery store and the bookstore for shopping. Dylan then started smiling more at patients and then spoke to a wonder man who would always acknowledge Dylan, even when he didn't open his eyes or speak back. These were all small improvements, and we knew we were in the right place. I knew from talking with a Spero mom prior to coming that we had to be patient and that it took time for the body to heal from the inside out. That was the hard part. We had waited so long to get our boy back, we wanted it so badly. Every day, we saw true miracles happening right in front of us. I was told by a Spero employee who was once a patient herself that first you see the healing happening, then you start to believe it can happen to you, and then you do it yourself. That is exactly what happened to our son.

Week seven, Dylan started to swallow for the first time in two years in cold laser therapy, and then when he went to his NMR therapy, he started to move his arms. His body was starting to wake up and heal. That weekend, Dylan ate and swallowed all of the food he put in his mouth, and he even wheeled himself around the parking lot and the movie theater. On Monday, August 26, just two months after arriving at Spero, Dylan started to walk. The start of week eight was the beginning of a second chance at life for our son. That Monday morning, Dylan could move all of his upper body, write on his own, and started to move his toes in his first therapy. Dr. K came to visit Dylan in his first therapy and told him how proud she was of him. We were all in tears, but you could see the determination in my son's eyes. He believed it now, and he was going to heal and live life again. That afternoon, we left in our van for lunch like we always did and went to our favorite fast-food restaurant drive-through. In the drive-through, Dylan said my legs are moving, and I think I can stand up. His dad said how do you know if you don't try! So Dylan unbuckled his wheelchair lap belt and seatbelt and stood up (the best he could in a van). We all started screaming, and everyone in the drive-through thought we were crazy. When we arrived back at the RV, instead of my husband wheeling him out and carrying him into the RV, Dylan walked out of the van on his own! He was a little rusty while walking because it had been over two years. But he did it. He walked around outside, went into the RV, put on his tennis shoes, tied them, went to the bathroom on his own, and washed his own hands. He was all smiles and so happy, something we had not seen in a long time. That night, Dylan pulled out the feeding tube that he had had in for two years. What a joy to see!

When we returned to Spero, Dylan stepped out of the van from the front seat (they kicked mom to the back seat), and one of his therapists saw him and ran to him, hugged him, and started to cry. We all walked into the clinic where everyone, patients, doctors, and therapists, celebrated his huge accomplishment. Others said he was an inspiration to them to keep going, which meant so much to Dylan. The clinic was just so uplifting and encouraging, and that gave Dylan the determination to completely heal. Then the next day, Dylan reached 100 in NMR therapy and joined the 100 CLUB! Which is very hard to do, especially since before that day, Dylan hadn't gone over 30.

By September 9th, just 10 weeks after starting at Spero, we were sitting in the waiting room at the end of the day after his NMR therapy, and Dylan looked at me so calmly and said, "Wow, that's weird, it's like all my pain just rushed out of my body." He was at ZERO pain for the first time in three years. Once again, everyone celebrated his win! By this time, as a family, we had gone out to a restaurant to eat dinner. That was such an amazing sight to see our son sitting in a restaurant, ordering dinner, talking to people, and eating dinner. Something you tend to take for granted. We rented electric scooters and rode them all around Fatteville. We had a blast. It was so much fun just enjoying life again. We also met some friends at Spero and went to dinner and the arcade with them.

Now Dylan's goals were to walk normally, run, and jump. He was determined to accomplish this goal. At the beginning of our journey, Spero had estimated 16 weeks for Dylan to graduate, and he did it in 15 weeks. He had been pain-free for 5 weeks and had accomplished his goals of walking without a limp, running, and jumping. His doctor set a graduation date for October 10th, 2024.

That was a huge day. Dylan was one of three to graduate that day. Another Long Covid patient also graduated with Dylan, a man with whom we had become close. Dylan and he had shared very dark and personal stories in therapy about the low points of their illness. They helped each other in ways they will never know. Graduation Day was full of amazing stories, smiles, tears, and most of all love! We were so blessed to have found Spero and met the amazing doctors, therapists, staff, and patients. They will forever be in our hearts and be our family.

Our journey home was much different than our journey to Arkansas. We took our time driving home and enjoyed camping as a family in the beautiful fall weather. We arrived home on October 19th, 2024, with Dylan's grandmothers waiting for us with open arms. Dylan had not seen or talked to them in almost two years because of his illness. He jumped out of the RV and hugged and kissed them both. There was a big, beautiful WELCOME HOME sign, cookies baking, lots of smiles, love, and a beautiful, clean house. Our mothers had taken care of our home as if it were their own. And let's not forget our cat Lily, whom they had taken care of for 4 months. She was so happy to see us, especially Dylan.

From November to January, we had Dylan tutored in math so that he could return to high school (9th grade). Dylan returned to school in January of his 9th-grade year. He has just completed his 9th grade year completely healthy and with straight A's. He was able to go to his high school Valentine's Dance (with a date) and rejoined his friends. This summer, he will be taking driver's ed and playing soccer in August for his sophomore year. Thank you to Dr. K, all the doctors, therapists, staff, and patients at Spero, you all have truly blessed our family! Spero saved our son's life!

Stacey Smith (Dylan's Mom)

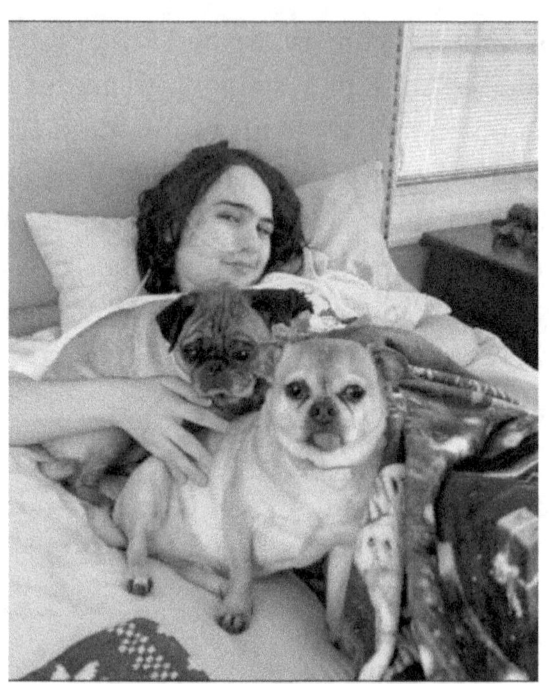

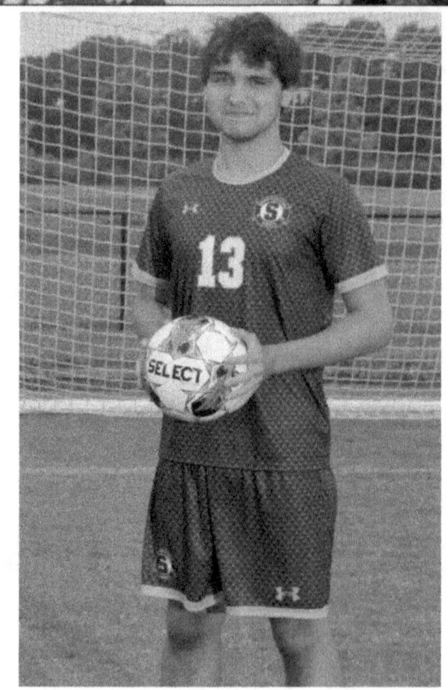

Chapter 10: Our system

B.J. Palmer

"The nervous system holds the key to the body's incredible potential to heal itself."

J. Holder

A Strategic Approach to Pediatric Long COVID Recovery

At The Spero Clinic, we recognize that Long COVID in children is not only real—it is profoundly life-altering. Fatigue, brain fog, pain, heart rate irregularities, and a host of other confusing, often invisible symptoms can turn a thriving child into a shell of who they once were. As a parent, you're likely exhausted, frightened, and out of options. That's where we come in—with a strategic system designed to treat the whole child, not just a list of symptoms.

We don't operate from guesswork or temporary symptom relief. Our system is rooted in clinical clarity and driven by outcomes. Using a precise, individualized roadmap built from advanced neurological, metabolic, and autonomic diagnostics, we uncover what is truly happening beneath the surface. From there, we execute a custom, full-body treatment program focused on recalibrating and restoring your child's nervous system, cellular health, and immune resilience.

Long COVID is complex. But so is our system. That's intentional.

We combine the best of functional neurology, cellular rehabilitation, frequency therapy, nervous system re-integration, and cutting-edge supportive therapies—all delivered in a daily, structured format within a clinical setting. We focus on the why behind your child's suffering, not just the what. Our goal is to rebuild from the inside out, giving your child the tools to recover fully, naturally, and sustainably. Research has proven that if a medical team collaborates, patients do better. We therefore place a high value on collaboration and regularly meet as a team to discuss your child's case and treatment plan in detail.

This is not a one-size-fits-all or short-term solution. It is a highly personalized, high-accountability program built for families who are ready to take bold action. We collaborate closely with you every step of the way—evaluating, refining, and adapting care as your child progresses. Most importantly, we never lose sight of your child's potential.

Our mission is simple but bold: To help your child reclaim their life. If you've been told to "just wait it out," if your child has been dismissed or misdiagnosed, or if traditional medicine has run out of answers—we're ready to be your next step. We exist for the cases that don't fit in a box. And we know how to fight for a future that looks nothing like the past.

At The Spero Clinic, one of the most critical factors in our success lies not just in *what* we do—but *how* and *when* we do it. Each therapy we offer is powerful on its own, but when integrated into a cohesive, simultaneous care plan, their combined impact becomes exponentially greater. I often explain it like a rope-pulling competition: one person pulling alone can't win the match, no matter how strong they are. But when a team pulls together in sync, they create an unstoppable force. It's the same with our system. If patients attempt these therapies individually or in isolation, they often see little to no lasting benefit—because the body requires a synchronized, multi-system approach to truly heal.

One of the most unique and essential aspects of our system at The Spero Clinic is its deliberate duality—a carefully calibrated balance between gentleness and intensity. We've spent years perfecting a treatment model that honors this delicate dance. On one side, we have an entire pillar of care dedicated to keeping the nervous system calm, regulated, and out of "fight or flight" mode. This is crucial, especially in pediatric Long COVID patients whose bodies are already overwhelmed.

A dysregulated nervous system can sabotage even the most advanced therapies, so we use specific techniques to create a foundation of safety and calm. At the same time, the other pillar of our system is designed to challenge the body—pushing just enough to awaken dormant systems, retrain dysfunction, and trigger healing. Without this intensity, there is no transformation. But without calm, there is no capacity to receive it. When done in harmony, this dual approach becomes a powerful engine for recovery. It's a formula that took years of refinement, and it's a core reason why our outcomes are so consistently life-changing.

Long COVID is complex, affecting multiple systems at once—neurological, immune, digestive, cardiovascular. Our treatments are intentionally layered, sequenced, and timed to work in harmony. This synergy is where transformation happens. This is not accidental—it's the design. And it's why our patients, especially pediatric ones, begin to climb out of the deepest trenches of illness when everything else has failed.

Our System:

At The Spero Clinic, we don't just treat symptoms—we address the root causes of dysfunction caused by pediatric long COVID. Our system is built around a unique integrative model that brings together leading-edge therapies in a synchronized, supportive environment. Each therapy is carefully selected for its ability to regulate the nervous system, reduce systemic inflammation, and restore cellular health. But the true power of our program lies in how these treatments work together, magnifying each other's effects. It's like a team pulling in perfect harmony: each therapy is powerful alone, but together they generate exponential healing. Here's how we do it:

Vagus Nerve Therapy

The vagus nerve is a vital communication highway between the brain and body. Long COVID often leads to autonomic nervous system (ANS) dysregulation, leaving children stuck in a state of fight or flight. Our gentle, patented manual technique applied to the upper cervical spine stimulates the vagus nerve, helping shift the body back into a healing, parasympathetic state. This activation reduces systemic inflammation, improves heart rate variability, regulates digestion, and helps rebalance immune and hormonal functions. Children often feel calmer, more emotionally regulated, and better able to engage in healing once this pathway is restored.

Magnetic Resonance Therapy (MRT)

MRT uses a full-body, low-intensity electromagnetic field to deliver targeted resonance to tissues based on their molecular structure. This therapy is particularly effective for children with chronic inflammation and cellular dysfunction. By normalizing electrical signaling in the body, MRT promotes improved blood flow, oxygenation, and nutrient delivery. It prepares tissues for deeper repair and primes the nervous system to respond more effectively to other treatments. For pediatric long COVID patients, this therapy helps calm the immune system and reduce symptoms like chronic fatigue and brain fog.

Pelvic Wave technology

The Pelvic Wave is a non-invasive neuromodulation therapy designed to stimulate the sacral nerves and pelvic region, which offers unique benefits for children with Long COVID. This gentle therapy works by improving communication between the nervous system and key organs involved in digestion, circulation, and autonomic regulation—all systems often disrupted in pediatric Long COVID. By activating the parasympathetic nervous system, Pelvic Wave may help reduce symptoms such as fatigue, brain fog, gastrointestinal issues, and poor circulation. It also supports vagus nerve tone, which plays a central role in calming inflammation and restoring homeostasis in the body. Because it is painless and requires no medication, Pelvic Wave can be a child-friendly option to include in a broader integrative recovery plan, especially for children experiencing nervous system dysregulation or POTS-like symptoms.

Microcurrent therapy

Microcurrent therapy is a gentle, non-invasive treatment that uses extremely low levels of electrical current—so low that most children don't feel anything at all. These currents are designed to mimic the body's own natural electrical signals, helping to "reboot" and support areas of the body that are struggling to heal. One of the biggest benefits of microcurrent therapy is that it helps the body produce more ATP, which is the main energy source for cells. For children with Long COVID, whose bodies may feel constantly tired or inflamed, this extra cellular energy can make a real difference in how they recover.

We've seen microcurrent therapy help ease muscle aches, calm irritated nerves, and speed up healing in tissues affected by inflammation or lack of blood flow. It's also gentle enough to use for a wide range of symptoms—whether a child is dealing with joint pain, headaches, stomach issues, or brain fog. Because no two children are the same, we adjust the frequencies and settings based on what each child's body needs most. Over time, this therapy can help reset the nervous system, reduce pain, and restore better function—giving children a safe and effective way to move forward in their healing.

Neuromuscular Re-Education

Children with long COVID often develop abnormal movement patterns due to pain, weakness, or nervous system dysfunction. Using FDA-approved bioelectric technology, this therapy retrains the body to move correctly. Unlike traditional physical therapy, which can take months to show results, neuromuscular re-education accelerates recovery by reestablishing proper communication between the brain and muscles. Children quickly regain strength, coordination, and confidence in their physical abilities, which plays a crucial role in their emotional and mental recovery as well.

Pelvic Wave Neuromuscular Stimulation Therapy

At The Spero Clinic, we use an advanced, FDA-cleared bio-electric magnet therapy—known as Pelvic Wave Therapy—to support neuromuscular rehabilitation in children affected by Long COVID. This non-invasive treatment stimulates tissue up to four inches deep without any skin contact, making it ideal for pediatric use. While originally developed and validated in over 44 clinical studies for pelvic floor rehabilitation, its applications extend to strengthening and reprogramming broader neuromuscular function.

This therapy works by delivering targeted magnetic pulses that cause involuntary muscle contractions. Unlike traditional exercise or physical therapy, these contractions are neurologically driven and help rebuild communication between the brain and muscles—creating new motor pathways and enhancing neuromuscular coordination. For children who have experienced neurological dysfunction, weakness, or motor control issues as a result of Long COVID, this therapy offers a powerful way to "re-educate" the nervous system.

The neuromuscular system governs every voluntary movement, relying on a precise dialogue between motor neurons and muscle fibers. Pelvic Wave Therapy facilitates this connection by activating the neuromuscular junction—where nerves and muscles meet—and triggering chemical signals that instruct muscles to contract. This process helps restore strength, stability, and functional movement, contributing to long-term rehabilitation and improved quality of life for pediatric patients.

Scar Tissue Therapy

Scar tissue, even when small or internal, can disrupt nerve signaling and lymphatic drainage. Scar therapy is not only caused by wounds or surgeries, but also by years of poor biomechanics and lack of movement. An unhealthy body that is often in pain will frequently develop unhealthy fascia. We use targeted soundwave therapy to gently break down these adhesions, restoring normal function and communication in the body. This is especially important in pediatric long COVID patients who have had surgeries, injuries, or chronic inflammation that could lead to hidden restrictions in tissues. This therapy improves range of motion, reduces pain, and removes one more barrier to total healing.

At The Spero Clinic, we use shock wave therapy as part of our integrative approach to treating pediatric Long COVID because of its powerful ability to stimulate healing at the cellular level without being invasive or painful. This therapy uses focused acoustic waves—delivered through a piezoelectric crystal—to trigger a biological response in damaged or inflamed tissues. In children suffering from Long COVID, where lingering inflammation, impaired circulation, and tissue dysfunction are common, Piezo shock waves can promote regeneration by increasing blood flow, reducing chronic pain, breaking up fascial restrictions, and encouraging the repair of soft tissues and nerves. Importantly, Piezo therapy is exceptionally precise and gentle, making it safe and well-tolerated in pediatric patients. By activating the body's natural healing mechanisms it helps restore function and reduce long-term complications in children whose systems have been destabilized by post-viral illness.

Low-Intensity Electrical Stimulation

This therapy uses gentle electrical impulses to calm irritated nerves, increase blood flow, and restore normal muscle tone. It is particularly effective for children suffering from neuropathic pain, muscle spasms, or sensory hypersensitivities. By reducing pain and improving tissue function, children can participate more fully in active therapies and regain lost functions faster. It's also an excellent tool to gently reintroduce healthy movement to areas that are guarded due to chronic pain.

Brain-and Body-Based Cold Laser Rehabilitation

Low-Level Laser Therapy (LLLT), also called cold laser therapy, is a safe and gentle treatment that uses low-intensity light to help heal and restore the brain and body. For children with Long COVID, certain parts of the brain—like those responsible for memory, attention, mood, and how the gut and brain communicate—can be slowed down or inflamed. Cold laser therapy targets these areas by shining a special light that helps support the mitochondria, which are tiny parts of cells that produce energy. This boost in energy helps the brain work better and heal faster.

The therapy also helps reduce inflammation in the brain, calming the "brain fog" and other symptoms like anxiety or mood swings that many kids experience after COVID. Another important benefit is that it encourages neuroplasticity—the brain's ability to reorganize and form new connections—which is key for recovering cognitive skills like focus, problem-solving, and emotional control. The treatment is completely non-invasive and pain-free, and because it is highly targeted, it focuses exactly on the brain regions that need help most. Many children notice improvements in their concentration, mood, and overall thinking abilities after a series of sessions, making this a promising option to include in a comprehensive care plan for pediatric Long COVID.

Hypnotherapy

Hypnotherapy is a helpful and gentle tool for children with Long COVID, especially when symptoms like fatigue, pain, anxiety, or trouble sleeping are present. Long COVID disrupts your child's nervous system, keeping their body in a constant state of stress that makes it harder to feel better. Hypnotherapy uses calming stories, guided imagery, and positive suggestions to help children relax deeply and feel safe in their own bodies again. In this relaxed state, the brain can shift from "fight-or-flight" mode into a healing state, supporting better sleep, reduced discomfort, and improved mood. For children, hypnotherapy often feels like guided daydreaming or play, making it both accessible and enjoyable. While it's not a standalone cure, it is a valuable part of a broader care plan—especially for children who feel overwhelmed or stuck in their recovery.

Ionic Detox Therapy

This therapy is incorporated as part of our program to support children battling Long COVID, a condition that often impairs the body's natural detoxification processes. This therapy works by rebalancing the body's cellular electrical charge, enhancing its ability to flush out toxins and inflammatory waste. During treatment, children comfortably place their feet in a specialized ionic footbath, where charged particles attract and neutralize harmful substances, drawing them out gently through the skin. Beyond detoxification, Ionic Therapy stimulates lymphatic flow, reduces swelling, helps maintain optimal pH balance, and increases overall energy levels. It is especially valuable for pediatric patients experiencing chronic fatigue, digestive discomfort, and weakened immune function, helping to restore vitality and support long-term recovery.

Neuromodulation

This gentle, non-invasive therapy helps recalibrate nerve signaling and restore balance to the autonomic nervous system. Using sophisticated electrical patterns, the therapy downregulates hypersensitive nerves and retrains them to interpret sensory input correctly. For pediatric patients experiencing sensory overload, chronic pain, or dysautonomia, neuromodulation can be a game-changer. It fosters nervous system resilience and brings lasting calm to children overwhelmed by their symptoms.

Customized Dietary Adjustments

No two children have the same biological makeup. We analyze food sensitivity testing and comprehensive blood analysis to design individualized nutrition plans. These adjustments address inflammation, gut dysfunction, and nutrient deficiencies commonly seen in pediatric long COVID. With the right diet in place, the body has the tools it needs to build new tissue, regulate the immune system, and maintain steady energy throughout the day. This is not a one-size-fits-all diet—it's a precision healing plan built just for them.

Blood Analysis

We perform in-depth laboratory testing to identify chronic infections, inflammation markers, hormonal imbalances, and nutritional deficiencies. Our clinical team has extensive experience recognizing patterns that conventional medicine often overlooks. The insights gained allow us to build a clear, actionable plan of care. It also helps us track progress and make timely adjustments, ensuring we stay aligned with each child's evolving needs.

Brain Balancing

Chronic illness disrupts brain function in ways that affect mood, sleep, behavior, and cognition. Brain balancing uses neurofeedback, vestibular input, and sensory integration exercises to restore healthy neural patterns. This therapy calms an overactive brain, improves emotional regulation, and helps reset disrupted circadian rhythms. It supports resilience in children who feel stuck, anxious, or mentally foggy, giving them back the focus and confidence they need to re-engage with life.

Oxygen Therapy

Oxygen therapy is an important part of our program. Oxygen is essential for life, but many children with Long COVID have trouble absorbing and using oxygen efficiently at the cellular level, which can lead to ongoing fatigue and difficulty thinking clearly. Our oxygen therapy uses carefully guided sessions of brief oxygen deprivation followed by reoxygenation to train the body to use oxygen better. This process helps improve how the heart and lungs work together to deliver oxygen throughout the body, making the cardiovascular system stronger and more efficient.

As a result, children often experience clearer thinking, better focus, and more energy to get through their day. For kids dealing with brain fog or overwhelming tiredness, this therapy can provide a noticeable boost in stamina and mental sharpness. The treatment is gentle, safe, and tailored to each child's unique needs, helping their body relearn how to maximize oxygen use for healing and recovery. Oxygen therapy is a valuable part of a complete Long COVID care plan, supporting both physical endurance and cognitive function.

Lymphatic therapy

This gentle, non-invasive treatment uses gentle resistance generated by special gases to encourage the body's lymphatic system to work more efficiently as a bulb filled with these gases is glided over the lymphatic system. The lymphatic system is like the body's natural drainage and cleaning network—it helps remove waste, toxins, and excess fluid from tissues. When this system becomes sluggish, waste and inflammation can build up, making it harder for the immune system to function properly.

Many children with Long COVID experience persistent inflammation and immune system challenges that can cause symptoms like fatigue, joint pain, and swelling. Lymphatic therapy helps by gently stimulating the lymph vessels to drain more effectively, which reduces fluid buildup and helps flush out toxins that may be fueling these symptoms. The therapy also supports a healthier immune response, giving the body a better chance to fight off lingering inflammation and infection.

Children who receive lymphatic therapy often report feeling lighter, less achy, and clearer mentally. This therapy can help restore balance and resilience to their bodies, making it an important tool in comprehensive Long COVID care. Because it's painless and relaxing, it's well-suited for kids and can be tailored to meet each child's specific needs.

The Power of Integration

The power of integration is what makes The Spero Clinic different. It isn't just the individual therapies we offer—it's how we bring them all together in a way that feels natural, thoughtful, and deeply personalized for each child. Imagine an orchestra warming up before a big performance: each instrument tuning itself, each musician finding their rhythm.

When they all come together, playing in harmony, the music transforms from noise into something beautiful and powerful. That's exactly how we approach healing. Every therapy, every treatment has its moment, its purpose, and when combined carefully, they create a healing "symphony" that speaks directly to your child's unique needs.

We understand that healing from Long COVID, especially in children, is not simple or straightforward. It's not about a quick fix or a single magic treatment. It's about supporting the body in the right way, at the right time—so the nervous system can relax, the immune system can rebuild, and the body can start to repair itself naturally. We have seen time and again that when the nervous system feels calm and safe, the body responds with less inflammation, less pain, and more energy. And when the immune system feels supported—not pushed or overwhelmed—it can better fight off lingering symptoms and restore balance.

Each therapy we use is carefully chosen and scheduled to work alongside the others, so they don't compete or conflict but instead build on each other's strengths. This layering effect means progress is not just possible—it becomes lasting. We don't just want to help your child feel better today; we want to help your child reclaim their life, their joy, and their future. Healing is a journey, sometimes slow and sometimes frustrating, but it is always possible. And when therapies are integrated thoughtfully, that journey becomes smoother and filled with hope.

At The Spero Clinic, we don't just treat symptoms. We treat your child as a whole person—body, mind, and spirit. We believe that every child has an incredible capacity to heal, grow, and thrive when given the right support. We are here to walk

beside you, offering not just treatments, but encouragement
and belief in your child's ability to overcome. Together, we can
create the conditions for real transformation—one step, one
therapy, one day at a time. Your child's healing story is still
being written, and with the power of integration, that story can
be one of hope, strength, and renewed life.

Guiding Principles for Parents

1. **Build a Support System** – Seek out professionals and
   positive support groups that understand long COVID.

2. **Remove Negativity** – Surround yourself and your child
   with encouragement and hope.

3. **No Apologies** – Your child's health challenges are not
   their fault, nor yours. Focus on progress, not guilt.

4. **Learn from Others** – Connect with families who have
   navigated long COVID recovery successfully.

5. **Be Your Child's Advocate** – Research treatments,
   question doctors, and make informed decisions.

6. **Stay Informed** – Use resources like Google Scholar to
   stay up-to-date on the latest research.

7. **Acknowledge the Reality** – Your child's condition is
   serious. Educate loved ones to foster understanding and
   support.

8. **Expect Recovery** – Keep hope alive. Mindset is a
   powerful factor in healing.

9. **Understand the Body's Systems** – Recognize the
   connection between different functions and promote
   holistic healing.

10. **Prioritize Wellness** – Ensure proper nutrition, hydration, and stress management.

11. **Activate the Parasympathetic Nervous System** – Encourage daily relaxation techniques like deep breathing and meditation.

12. **Maintain Social Connections** – Even small interactions can make a big difference in mental and emotional well-being.

13. **Be Open-Minded About Healthcare** – Effective treatment may come from various disciplines beyond conventional medicine.

14. **Demand Respectful Medical Care** – Work with compassionate, knowledgeable professionals who take your child's symptoms seriously.

Final Thoughts

You are not alone, and you are not wrong for fighting as hard as you are. What you're doing—advocating, researching, pushing for answers—takes immense strength, even when you feel like you're barely holding on. Your child is lucky to have you in their corner, and no matter how unseen or dismissed you may feel at times, your voice and your persistence matter deeply.

Long COVID in children is real, and it's devastating. It can feel like you're navigating a world that doesn't yet understand, with systems that aren't moving fast enough. But progress is being made—research is growing, more clinicians are listening, and communities of parents like you are reshaping what care looks like. Your determination is part of that change.

Right now, your job is to keep showing up. Not perfectly, not without exhaustion or tears—but with love and fierce resolve. Celebrate even the smallest steps forward. Rest when you can, cry when you need to, and then get back up. Build a team of people who believe your child's story. Keep learning, questioning, and trusting your instincts.

Your child doesn't need perfection—they need your presence, your belief in their future, and your unwavering refusal to give up. That kind of hope is healing in itself.

You're not just fighting for your child's survival. You're helping pave the way for their recovery. That matters more than words can say. And you don't have to do it alone—there are people, resources, and support ready to stand with you. Let's keep going, together.

Your child's journey with long COVID does not define their future—it is a chapter, not the whole story. The human body is astonishing in its resilience, and with the right guidance, patience, and care, healing is not only possible—it is likely. What may feel like a detour today can become the path to a deeper understanding of strength, perseverance, and the power of love. As parents, your advocacy, your belief, and your refusal to give up are lifelines your child can hold onto as they fight their way back to health. Keep asking questions. Keep seeking answers. Keep showing up. You are not alone, and neither are they.

"Although the world is full of suffering, it is also full of the overcoming of it."

— **Helen Keller**

The End

References

Chapter 1

1. Eccles, J. A., Cadar, D., Quadt, L., Hakim, A. J., Gall, N., Consortium, C. S. S. B., Bowyer, V., Cheetham, N., Steves, C. J., Critchley, H. D., & Davies, K. A. (2024, March 19). *Is joint hypermobility linked to self-reported non-recovery from COVID-19? Case–control evidence from the British covid symptom study Biobank.* BMJ Public Health. https://bmjpublichealth.bmj.com/content/2/1/e000478

2. Klein, J., Wood, J., Jaycox, J. R., Dhodapkar, R., Lu, P., Gehlhausen, J., Tabachnikova, A., Greene, K., Tabacof, L., Malik, A., Monteiro, V., Silva, J., Kamath, K., Zhang, M., Dhal, A., Ott, I., Valle, G., Peña-Hernández, M., Mao, T., ... Iwasaki, A. (2023, September 25). *Distinguishing features of long Covid identified through immune profiling.* Nature. https://pubmed.ncbi.nlm.nih.gov/37748514/

3. Buonsenso, D., Munblit, D., De Rose, C., Sinatti, D., Ricchiuto, A., Carfi, A., & Valentini, P. (2021, July). *Preliminary evidence on Long Covid in children.* Acta paediatrica (Oslo, Norway : 1992). https://pubmed.ncbi.nlm.nih.gov/33835507/

4. Smith, C., Odd, D., Harwood, R., Ward, J., Linney, M., Clark, M., Hargreaves, D., Ladhani, S., Draper, E., Viner, R., & Fraser, L. (2022, January 28). *Deaths in children and young people in England after SARS-COV-2 infection during the first pandemic year.* Nature medicine. https://pubmed.ncbi.nlm.nih.gov/34764489/

5. Guerrerio, A. L., Mateja, A., MacCarrick, G., Fintzi, J., Brittain, E., Frischmeyer-Guerrerio, P. A., & Dietz, H. C.

(2024). Web-based survey investigating cardiovascular complications in hypermobile Ehlers-Danlos syndrome after COVID-19 infection and vaccination. *PLOS ONE*, *19*(3), e0298272. https://doi.org/10.1371/journal.pone.0298272

6. Al-Aly, Z., Bowe, B., & Xie, Y. (2022). Long-term cardiovascular outcomes of COVID-19. *Nature Medicine*, *28*(3), 583–590. https://doi.org/10.1038/s41591-022-01689-3

    PMCID: PMC8926393 | PMID: 35257802

7. Antonelli, M., Pujol, J. C., Spector, T. D., Ourselin, S., & Steves, C. J. (2022). Risk of long COVID associated with delta versus omicron variants of SARS-CoV-2. *The Lancet Respiratory Medicine*. Advance online publication. https://www.thelancet.com/article/S1473-3099(21)00460-6/fulltext

8. Patterson, B. K., Yogendra, R., Francisco, E. B., Guevara-Coto, J., Long, E., Pise, A., Osgood, E., Bream, J., Kreimer, M., Jeffers, D., Beaty, C., Vander Heide, R., & Mora-Rodríguez, R. A. (2025). Detection of S1 spike protein in CD16+ monocytes up to 245 days in SARS-CoV-2-negative post-COVID-19 vaccine syndrome (PCVS) individuals. *Human Vaccines & Immunotherapeutics*, *21*(1), 2494934.https://doi.org/10.1080/21645515.2025.2494934

9. Yin, K., Peluso, M. J., Luo, X., Thomas, R., Shin, M., Neidleman, J., Andrew, A., Young, K. C., Ma, T., Hoh, R., Anglin, K., Huang, B., Argueta, U., Lopez, M., Valdivieso, D., Asare, K., Deveau, T., Munter, S. E., Ibrahim, R., Ständker, L., Lu, S., Goldberg, S. A., Lee, S. A., Lynch, K. L., Kelly, J. D., Martin, J. N., Münch, J., Deeks, S. G., Henrich, T. J., & Roan, N. R. (2024). Long COVID manifests with T

cell dysregulation, inflammation, and an uncoordinated adaptive immune response to SARS-CoV-2. *Nature Immunology, 25,* 218–225. https://pubmed.ncbi.nlm.nih.gov/38212464/

PMCID: PMC10284676 | PMID: 37628107

10. Lei, Y., Zhang, J., Schiavon, C. R., He, M., Chen, L., Shen, H., ... Wu, H. (2021). SARS-CoV-2 spike protein impairs endothelial function via downregulation of ACE2. *Circulation Research, 128*(9), 1323–1326. https://doi.org/10.1161/CIRCRESAHA.121.318902

PMCID: PMC8457363 | PMID: 33846854

11. Yonker, L. M., Swank, Z., Bartsch, Y. C., Burns, M. D., Kane, A., Boribong, B. P., Davis, J. P., Loiselle, M., Novak, T., Senussi, Y., Cheng, C.-A., Burgess, E., Edlow, A. G., Chou, J., Dionne, A., Balaguru, D., Lahoud-Rahme, M., Arditi, M., Julg, B., Randolph, A. G., Alter, G., Fasano, A., & Walt, D. R. (2023). Circulating spike protein detected in post–COVID-19 mRNA vaccine myocarditis. *Circulation, 147*(11), 867–876. https://doi.org/10.1161/CIRCULATIONAHA.122.061025

PMCID: PMC9876790 | PMID: 36551048

12. Boros, L. G., Kyriakopoulos, A. M., Brogna, C., Piscopo, M., McCullough, P. A., & Seneff, S. (2024). Long-lasting, biochemically modified mRNA, and its frameshifted recombinant spike proteins in human tissues and circulation after COVID-19 vaccination. *Pharmacology Research & Perspectives, 12*(3), e1218. https://doi.org/10.1002/prp2.1218

PMCID: PMC11169277 PMID: 38867495

13. Röltgen, K., et al. (2022). Immune imprinting, breadth of variant recognition, and germinal center response in human SARS-CoV-2 infection and vaccination. *Cell, 185*(6), 1025–1040.e14. https://doi.org/10.1016/j.cell.2022.01.018

14. Conti, V., Corbi, G., Sabbatino, F., De Pascale, D., Sellitto, C., Stefanelli, B., Bertini, N., De Simone, M., Liguori, L., Di Paola, I., De Bernardo, M., Tesse, A., Rosa, N., Pagliano, P., & Filippelli, A. (2023). Long COVID: Clinical framing, biomarkers, and therapeutic approaches. *Journal of Personalized Medicine, 13*(2), 334. https://doi.org/10.3390/jpm13020334

PMCID: PMC9959656 | PMID: 36836568

15. Rathod, N., Kumar, S., Chavhan, R., Acharya, S., & Rathod, S. (2024). Navigating the long haul: A comprehensive review of long-COVID sequelae, patient impact, pathogenesis, and management. *Cureus, 16*(5), e60176. https://doi.org/10.7759/cureus.60176

PMCID: PMC11167581 | PMID: 38868283

Chapter 3

1. Lorman, V., Bailey, L. C., Song, X., Rao, S., Hornig, M., Utidjian, L., Razzaghi, H., Mejias, A., Leikauf, J. E., Brill, S. B., Allen, A., Bunnell, H. T., Reedy, C., Mosa, A. S. M., Horne, B. D., Geary, C. R., Chuang, C. H., Williams, D. A., Christakis, D. A., & Forrest, C. B.(2024, September 18). *Pediatric long COVID subphenotypes: An EHR-based study from the RECOVER program* [Preprint]. medRxiv. https://pmc.ncbi.nlm.nih.gov/articles/PMC11451761/

2. Lorman, V., Bailey, L. C., Song, X., Rao, S., Hornig, M., Utidjian, L., Razzaghi, H., Mejias, A., Leikauf, J. E., Brill, S.

B., Allen, A., Bunnell, H. T., Reedy, C., Mosa, A. S. M., Horne, B. D., Reynolds Geary, C., Chuang, C. H., Williams, D. A., Christakis, D. A., … Forrest, C. B. (2024, September 18). *Pediatric long COVID subphenotypes: An EHR-based study from the RECOVER program* [Preprint]. medRxiv. https://doi.org/10.1101/2024.09.17.24313742

3. Henning E;Musci R;Johnson SB;Villatoro C;Malone LA;, E., Musci, R., Johnson, S., Villatoro, C., & Malone, L. (2025, May 6). *Pediatric long covid: Relationships with premorbid history of anxiety or depression and health-related quality of life*. Journal of Pediatric Psychology. https://pubmed.ncbi.nlm.nih.gov/40327758/

4. Vaz, A;Costa, A;Pinto, A;Silva, A. I;Figueiredo, P;Sarmento, A;& Santos, L. (2021). Complex regional pain syndrome after severe COVID-19 – A case report. *Heliyon, 7*(11), e08462. https://doi.org/10.1016/j.heliyon.2021.e08462

5. Shehab, D., Abdulsalam, A. J., & Reebye, R. N. (2022). Complex regional pain syndrome as a sequela of COVID-19 pneumonia. *Revue Neurologique, 178*(8), 865–867. https://doi.org/10.1016/j.neurol.2022.03.013

6. Zollinger, P. E., Tuinebreijer, W. E., Breederveld, R. S., & Kreis, R. W. (2007). Can vitamin C prevent complex regional pain syndrome in patients with wrist fractures? A randomized, controlled, multicenter dose-response study. *The Journal of Bone and Joint Surgery. American Volume, 89*(7), 1424–1431. https://pubmed.ncbi.nlm.nih.gov/17606778/

7. Raj, S. R., Arnold, A. C., Barboi, A., Claydon, V. E., Limberg, J. K., Lucci, V. M., … & Vernino, S. (2021). Long-COVID postural tachycardia syndrome: An American

Autonomic Society statement. *Clinical Autonomic Research, 31*(3), 365–368. https://pubmed.ncbi.nlm.nih.gov/33740207/

8. Khurana, S., et al. (2022). Pediatric postural orthostatic tachycardia syndrome in long COVID: A review of clinical features and management. *Frontiers in Pediatrics, 10*, 848615. https://www.frontiersin.org/journals/cardiovascular-medicine/articles/10.3389/fcvm.2022.860198/full

9. Castori, M., Tinkle, B., Levy, H., Grahame, R., Malfait, F., & Hakim, A. (2017). A framework for the classification of joint hypermobility and related conditions. *American Journal of Medical Genetics Part C: Seminars in Medical Genetics, 175*(1), 148–157. https://doi.org/10.1002/ajmg.c.31545

10. Carmona-Torre, F., Minguez-Olaondo, A., Lopez-Bravo, A., Tijero, B., Grozeva, V., Walcker, M., Azkune-Galparsoro, H., Lopez de Munain, A., Alcaide, A. B., Quiroga, J., Pozo, J. L. del, & Gomez-Esteban, J. C. (2022, May 26). *Dysautonomia in COVID-19 patients: A narrative review on clinical course, Diagnostic and Therapeutic Strategies.* Frontiers. https://www.frontiersin.org/journals/neurology/articles/10.3389/fneur.2022.886609/full

11. Mavroudis, I., Kazis, D., Kamal, F. Z., Gurzu, I.-L., Ciobica, A., Pădurariu, M., Novac, B., & Iordache, A. (2024, April 18). *Understanding functional neurological disorder: Recent insights and diagnostic challenges.* International journal of molecular sciences. https://pmc.ncbi.nlm.nih.gov/articles/PMC11050230/

12. O'dor, S. L., Zagaroli, J., Belisle, R., Hamel, M., Downer, O., Homayoun, S., & Williams, K. (2022, August 5). *The COVID-19 pandemic and children with pans/Pandas: An evaluation of symptom severity, telehealth, and vaccination hesitancy - child psychiatry & human development.* Child Psychiatry and Human Development. https://link.springer.com/article/10.1007/s10578-022-01401-z

13. Berloffa, S., Salvati, A., Pantalone, G., Falcioni, L., Rizzi, M. M., Naldini, F., Masi, G., & Gagliano, A. (2023, February 14). *Steroid treatment response to post SARS-COV-2 pans symptoms: Case series.* Frontiers in Neurology. https://pubmed.ncbi.nlm.nih.gov/36864920/

14. Zhang, F., Lau, R. I., Liu, Q., Su, Q., Chan, F. K. L., & Ng, S. C. (2022, October 21). *Gut Microbiota in COVID-19: Key microbial changes, potential mechanisms and clinical applications.* Nature News. https://www.nature.com/articles/s41575-022-00698-4

15. Puoti, M. G., Rybak, A., Kiparissi, F., Gaynor, E., & Borrelli, O. (2021, February 21). *SARS-COV-2 and the gastrointestinal tract in children.* Frontiers. https://www.frontiersin.org/journals/pediatrics/articles/10.3389/fped.2021.617980/full

16. Bitar, R. R., Alattas, B., Azaz, A., Rawat, D., & Miqdady, M. (2022, December 20). *Gastrointestinal manifestations in children with covid-19 infection: Retrospective Tertiary Center Experience.* Frontiers. https://www.frontiersin.org/journals/pediatrics/articles/10.3389/fped.2022.925520/full

17. Dimino, J., & Kuo, B. (2025, April 5). *Current concepts in gastroparesis and gastric neuromuscular disorders-pathophysiology, diagnosis, and management*. MDPI. https://www.mdpi.com/2075-4418/15/7/935

18. Hakim, A. (2024, February 22). *Hypermobile Ehlers-Danlos syndrome*. GeneReviews® [Internet]. https://www.ncbi.nlm.nih.gov/books/NBK1279/

19. Castori, M., Tinkle, B., Levy, H., Grahame, R., Malfait, F., & Hakim, A. (2017, March 17). *A framework for the classification of joint hypermobility and related conditions*. American journal of medical genetics. Part C, Seminars in medical genetics. https://pubmed.ncbi.nlm.nih.gov/28145606/

20. Castori, M., Tinkle, B., Levy, H., Grahame, R., Malfait, F., & Hakim, A. (2017, March 17). *A framework for the classification of joint hypermobility and related conditions*. American journal of medical genetics. Part C, Seminars in medical genetics. https://pubmed.ncbi.nlm.nih.gov/28145606/

21. Blitshteyn, S., & Whitelaw, S. (2021, April 6). *Postural orthostatic tachycardia syndrome (POTS) and other autonomic disorders after COVID-19 infection: A case series of 20 patients*. Immunologic research. https://pubmed.ncbi.nlm.nih.gov/33786700/

22. Dani, M., Dirksen, A., Taraborrelli, P., Torocastro, M., Panagopoulos, D., Sutton, R., & Lim, P. B. (2021, January). *Autonomic dysfunction in "long covid": Rationale, physiology and Management Strategies*. Clinical medicine (London, England). https://pmc.ncbi.nlm.nih.gov/articles/PMC7850225/

23. Ganesh, R., & Munipalli, B. (2024, September 5). *Long Covid and hypermobility spectrum disorders have shared pathophysiology*. Frontiers in neurology. https://pmc.ncbi.nlm.nih.gov/articles/PMC11410636/#:~:text=Clinical%20features%20of%20hEDS%20include,to%20pain%20amplification%20(15).

24. Malfait, F., Francomano, C., Byers, P., Belmont, J., Berglund, B., Black, J., Bloom, L., Bowen, J., Brady, A., Burrows, N., Castori, M., Cohen, H., Colombi, M., Demirdas, S., De Backer, J., De Paepe, A., Fournel-Gigleux, S., Frank, M., Ghali, N., ... Tinkle, B. (2017, March 17). *The 2017 international classification of the ehlers–danlos syndromes - malfait - 2017 - American Journal of Medical Genetics Part C: Seminars in Medical Genetics - Wiley Online Library*. American journal of medical genetics Seminars in medical genetics Part C. https://onlinelibrary.wiley.com/doi/full/10.1002/ajmg.c.31552

25. Jason, L. A., Islam, M., Conroy, K., Cotler, J., Torres, C., Johnson, M., & Mabie, B. (2021, April 21). *Covid-19 symptoms over time: Comparing long-haulers to me/CFS*. American ME and CFS Society. https://www.tandfonline.com/doi/full/10.1080/21641846.2021.1922140

26. Bosworth, M., Pawelek, P., & Ayoubkhani, D. (2023, January 5). *Prevalence of ongoing symptoms following coronavirus (COVID-19) infection in the UK: 5 january 2023*. Prevalence of ongoing symptoms following coronavirus (COVID-19) infection in the UK - Office for National Statistics. https://www.ons.gov.uk/peoplepopulationandcommunity

/healthandsocialcare/conditionsanddiseases/bulletins/pre
valenceofongoingsymptomsfollowingcoronaviruscovid19in
fectionintheuk/5january2023

27. Proal, A. D., & VanElzakker, M. B. (2021, June 22). *Long
Covid or post-acute sequelae of COVID-19 (PASC): An
overview of biological factors that may contribute to
persistent symptoms*. Frontiers.
https://frontiersin.org/articles/10.3389/fmicb.2021.698169/
full

Chapter 4

1. Cohn, L. N., Pechlivanoglou, P., Lee, Y., Mahant, S., Orkin, J., Marson, A., & Cohen, E. (2020). Health outcomes of parents of children with chronic illness: A systematic review and meta-analysis. *Journal of Pediatrics, 218*, 166–177.e2. https://doi.org/10.1016/j.jpeds.2019.10.068

2. Russell, B. S., Hutchison, M., Tambling, R., Tomkunas, A. J., & Horton, A. L. (2020). Initial challenges of caregiving during COVID-19: Caregiver burden, mental health, and the parent-child relationship. *Child Psychiatry & Human Development, 51*(5), 671–682. https://doi.org/10.1007/s10578-020-01037-x

Chapter 5

1. Williams, E. S., Martins, T. B., Shah, K. S., Hill, H. R., Coiras, M., Spivak, A. M., & Planelles, V. (2023, February 2). *Cytokine deficiencies in patients with long-COVID.* Journal of clinical & cellular immunology. https://pmc.ncbi.nlm.nih.gov/articles/PMC9894377/

2. Sarubbo, F., El Haji, K., Vidal-Balle, A., & Bargay Lleonart, J. (2022). Neurological consequences of COVID-19 and brain related pathogenic mechanisms: A new challenge for neuroscience. *Brain, Behavior, & Immunity - Health, 19*, 100399. https://doi.org/10.1016/j.bbih.2021.100399

3. Kong, Z., Wang, J., Li, T., Zhang, Z., & Jian, J. (2020). 2019 novel coronavirus pneumonia with onset of dizziness: A case report. *Annals of Translational Medicine, 8*(15), 1030. https://doi.org/10.21037/atm.2020.03.89

4. Hamming, I., Timens, W., Bulthuis, M. L. C., Lely, A. T., Navis, G. J., & van Goor, H. (2004). Tissue distribution of

ACE2 protein, the functional receptor for SARS coronavirus: A first step in understanding SARS pathogenesis. *The Journal of Pathology, 203*(2), 631–637. https://doi.org/10.1002/path.1570

5. Meinhardt, J., Radke, J., Dittmayer, C., Franz, J., Thomas, C., Mothes, R., Laue, M., Schneider, J., Brünink, S., Greuel, S., Lehmann, M., Hassan, O., Aschman, T., Schumann, E., Chua, R. L., Conrad, C., Eils, R., Stenzel, W., Windgassen, M., … Heppner, F. L. (2021). Olfactory transmucosal SARS-CoV-2 invasion as a port of central nervous system entry in individuals with COVID-19. *Nature Neuroscience, 24*(2), 168–175. https://doi.org/10.1038/s41593-020-00758-5

6. Lurie, I., Yang, Y.-X., Haynes, K., & Boursi, B. (2015, November 7). *Antibiotic exposure and the risk for depression, anxiety, or psychosis: A nested case-control study*. The Journal of clinical psychiatry. https://pubmed.ncbi.nlm.nih.gov/26580313/

7. Bellon, M., Schweblin, C., Lambeng, N., Cherpillod, P., Vazquez, J., Lalive, P. H., Schibler, M., & Deffert, C. (2021). Cerebrospinal fluid features in severe acute respiratory syndrome coronavirus 2 (SARS-CoV-2) reverse transcription polymerase chain reaction (RT-PCR) positive patients. *Clinical Infectious Diseases, 73*(6), e3102–e3105. https://doi.org/10.1093/cid/ciaa1165

8. Hernández-Parra, H., Reyes-Hernández, O. D., Figueroa-González, G., González-Del Carmen, M., González-Torres, M., Peña-Corona, S. I., Florán, B., Cortés, H., & Leyva-Gómez, G. (2023). Alteration of the blood-brain barrier by COVID-19 and its implication in the permeation of drugs

into the brain. *Frontiers in Cellular Neuroscience, 17,* 1125109. https://doi.org/10.3389/fncel.2023.1125109

9. Arbour, N., Côté, G., Lachance, C., Tardieu, M., Cashman, N. R., & Talbot, P. J. (1999). Acute and persistent infection of human neural cell lines by human coronavirus OC43. *Journal of Virology, 73*(4), 3338–3350. https://doi.org/10.1128/JVI.73.4.3338-3350.1999

10. Song, E., Zhang, C., Israelow, B., Lu-Culligan, A., Prado, A. V., Skriabine, S., Lu, P., Weizman, O.-E., Liu, F., Dai, Y., Szigeti-Buck, K., Yasumoto, Y., Wang, G., Castaldi, C., Heltke, J., Ng, E., Wheeler, J., Madel Alfajaro, M., Levavasseur, E., … Iwasaki, A. (2021, January 12). *Neuroinvasion of SARS-COV-2 in human and Mouse Brain | Journal of Experimental Medicine | Rockefeller University press.* Journal of Experimental Medicine. https://rupress.org/jem/article/218/3/e20202135/211674/Ne uroinvasion-of-SARS-CoV-2-in-human-and-mouse

11. Tian, M., et al. (2021). HIF-1α promotes SARS-CoV-2 infection and aggravates inflammatory responses to COVID-19. *Signal Transduction and Targeted Therapy, 6*(1), 308. https://doi.org/10.1038/s41392-021-00726-w

12. Kandemirli, S. G., Dogan, L., Sarikaya, Z. T., Kara, S., Akinci, C., Kaya, D., Kaya, Y., Yildirim, D., Tuzuner, F., Yildirim, M. S., Ozluk, E., Gucyetmez, B., Karaarslan, E., Koyluoglu, I., Demirel Kaya, H. S., Mammadov, O., Ozdemir, I. K., Afsar, N., Yalcinkaya, B. C., Rasimoglu, S., Guduk, D. E., Jima, A. K., Ilksoz, A., Ersoz, V., Eren, M. Y., Celtik, N., Arslan, S., Korkmazer, B., Dincer, S. S., Gulek, E., Dikmen, I., Yazici, M., Unsal, S., Ljama, T., Demirel, I., Ayyildiz, A., Kesimci, I., Deveci, S. B., Tutuncu, M.,

Kizilkilic, O., Telci, L., Zengin, R., Dincer, A., Akinci, I. O., & Kocer, N. (2020). Brain MRI findings in patients in the intensive care unit with COVID-19 infection. *Radiology*, 297(1), E232–E235. https://doi.org/10.1148/radiol.2020201697

13. Bernal, K. D. E., & Whitehurst, C. B. (2023). Incidence of Epstein-Barr virus reactivation is elevated in COVID-19 patients. *Virus Research*. Advance online publication. https://doi.org/10.1016/j.virusres.2023.199157

14. Merbouh, M., El Aidouni, G., Bkiyar, H., & Housni, B. (2023). Post COVID-19 trigeminal neuritis: Case report. *Radiology Case Reports*. Advance online publication. https://doi.org/10.1016/j.radcr.2023.04.051

15. Sasso, E. M., Muraki, K., Eaton-Fitch, N., Smith, P., Lesslar, O. L., Deed, G., & Marshall-Gradisnik, S. (2022, August 19). *Transient receptor potential melastatin 3 dysfunction in post covid-19 condition and myalgic encephalomyelitis/chronic fatigue syndrome patients - molecular medicine*. BioMed Central. https://molmed.biomedcentral.com/articles/

Chapter 6

1. Ali, S., Kang, A., Patel, T., Clark, J., Perez-Giraldi, G., Orban, Z., Lim, P., Jimenez, M., Graham, E., Batra, A., Liotta, E., & Koralnik, I. (2022, July). *Evolution of neurologic symptoms in non-hospitalized COVID-19 "long haulers" - northwestern scholars*. Northwestern Scholars Neurology. https://www.scholars.northwestern.edu/en/publications/evolution-of-neurologic-symptoms-in-non-hospitalized-covid-19-lon

2.   Ojeda, A., Calvo, A., Cuñat, T., Mellado-Artigas, R., Comino-Trinidad, O., Aliago, J., Arias, M., Ferrando, C., Martinez-Pallí, G., & Dürsteler, C. (2022, March 26). *Characteristics and influence on quality of life of new-onset pain in critical covid-19 survivors.* European journal of pain (London, England). https://pubmed.ncbi.nlm.nih.gov/34866276/

3.   Huang, C., Wang, Y., Li, X., Ren, L., Zhao, J., Hu, Y., et al. (2020). Clinical features of patients infected with 2019 novel coronavirus in Wuhan, China. *The Lancet, 395*(10223), 497–506. https://doi.org/10.1016/S0140-6736(20)30183-5

4.   del Valle, D. M., Kim-Schulze, S., Huang, H. H., Beckmann, N. D., Nirenberg, S., Wang, B., et al. (2020). An inflammatory cytokine signature predicts COVID-19 severity and survival. *Nature Medicine, 26*(10), 1636–1643. https://doi.org/10.1038/s41591-020-1051-9

5.   Lei, X., Dong, X., Ma, R., Wang, W., Xiao, X., Tian, Z., et al. (2020). Activation and evasion of type I interferon responses by SARS-CoV-2. *Nature Communications, 11*(1), 3810. https://doi.org/10.1038/s41467-020-17665-9

6.   Bayat, A.-H., Azimi, H., Hassani Moghaddam, M., Ebrahimi, V., Fathi, M., Vakili, K., Mahmoudiasl, G.-R., Forouzesh, M., Eskandarian Boroujeni, M., Nariman, Z., Abbaszadeh, H.-A., Aryan, A., Aliaghaei, A., & Abdollahifar, M.-A. (2022). COVID-19 causes neuronal degeneration and reduces neurogenesis in human hippocampus. *Apoptosis, 27*(11-12), 852–868. https://doi.org/10.1007/s10495-022-01754-9

7. Dubey, S., Das, S., Ghosh, R., Jana Dubey, M., Chakraborty, A. P., Roy, D., Das, G., Dutta, A., Santra, A., Sengupta, S., & Benito-León, J. (2023). The effects of SARS-CoV-2 infection on the cognitive functioning of patients with pre-existing dementia. *Journal of Alzheimer's Disease Reports, 7*(1), 119–128. https://doi.org/10.3233/ADR-220090

8. *Braga, J., Lepra, M., Kish, S. J., Rusjan, P. M., Nasser, Z., Verhoeff, N., Vasdev, N., Bagby, M., Boileau, I., Husain, M. I., Kolla, N., Garcia, A., Chao, T., Mizrahi, R., Faiz, K., Vieira, E. L., & Meyer, J. H. (2023). Neuroinflammation after COVID-19 with persistent depressive and cognitive symptoms. JAMA Psychiatry, 80(8), 787–795. https://doi.org/10.1001/jamapsychiatry.2023.1321*

9. Andrews, M. G., Mukhtar, T., Eze, U. C., Simone, A., Levantovsky, R., Salma, J., Karp, C., & Pleasure, S. J. (2022). Tropism of SARS-CoV-2 for human cortical astrocytes. *Proceedings of the National Academy of Sciences, 119*(29), e2122236119. https://doi.org/10.1073/pnas.2122236119

10. Pellegrini, L., Albecka, A., Mallery, D. L., Kowalski, L., Maini, P. K., McCoy, L. E., & Lancaster, M. A. (2020). SARS-CoV-2 infects the brain choroid plexus and disrupts the blood–CSF barrier in human brain organoids. *Cell Stem Cell, 27*(6), 951–961.e5. https://doi.org/10.1016/j.stem.2020.10.001

11. Shabani, Z. (2021). Demyelination as a result of an immune response in patients with COVID-19. *Acta Neurologica Belgica, 121*(4), 859–866. https://doi.org/10.1007/s13760-021-01691-5

12. Wei, Z.-Y. D., Liang, K., & Shetty, A. K. (2023). Role of microglia, decreased neurogenesis and oligodendrocyte depletion in Long COVID-mediated brain impairments. *Aging and Disease, 14*(6), 1958–1966. https://doi.org/10.14336/AD.2023.10918

13. Pan, R., Anthony, S., & Perlman, S. (2020, February 22). *Oligodendrocytes that survive acute coronavirus infection induce prolonged inflammatory responses in the CNS | PNAS*. PNAS. https://www.pnas.org/content/117/27/15902

14. Deffner, F., Scharr, M., Klingenstein, S., Klingenstein, M., Milazzo, A., Scherer, S., Wagner, A., Hirt, B., Mack, A. F., & Neckel, P. H. (2020). Histological evidence for the enteric nervous system and the choroid plexus as alternative routes of neuroinvasion by SARS-CoV2. *Frontiers in Neuroanatomy, 14*, 596439. https://doi.org/10.3389/fnana.2020.596439

15. Turner, M. D., Nedjai, B., Hurst, T., & Pennington, D. J. (2014). Cytokines and chemokines: At the crossroads of cell signalling and inflammatory disease. *Biochimica et Biophysica Acta (BBA) - Molecular Cell Research, 1843*(11), 2563–2582. https://doi.org/10.1016/j.bbamcr.2014.05.014

16. DiSabato, D. J., Quan, N., & Godbout, J. P. (2016). Neuroinflammation: The devil is in the details. *Journal of Neurochemistry, 139*(Suppl 2), 136–153. https://doi.org/10.1111/jnc.13607

Chapter 7

1. Lopez, J., & Tait, S. W. G. (2015, March 17). *Mitochondrial apoptosis: Killing cancer using the enemy within*. British journal of cancer.

https://www.ncbi.nlm.nih.gov/pmc/articles/PMC4366906/

2. Klein, K., He, K., Younes, A. I., Barsoumian, H. B., Chen, D., Ozgen, T., Mosaffa, S., Patel, R. R., Gu, M., Novaes, J., Narayanan, A., Cortez, M. A., & Welsh, J. W. (2020). Role of mitochondria in cancer immune evasion and potential therapeutic approaches. *Frontiers in Immunology, 11,* Article 573326. https://doi.org/10.3389/fimmu.2020.573326

3. Lyssiotis, C. (2017, June 9). *Powering off cancer.* RAS Initiative Blog. National Cancer Institute. https://www.cancer.gov/research/key-initiatives/ras/blog/2017/powering-off-cancer

4. Chen, T. H., Chang, C. J., & Hung, P. H. (2023). Possible pathogenesis and prevention of long COVID: SARS-CoV-2-induced mitochondrial disorder. *International Journal of Molecular Sciences, 24*(9), 8034. https://doi.org/10.3390/ijms24098034

5. Appelman, B., Charlton, B. T., Goulding, R. P., et al. (2024). Muscle abnormalities worsen after post-exertional malaise in long COVID. *Nature Communications, 15,* 17. https://doi.org/10.1038/s41467-023-44432-3

6. Ozturk, A., Bayraktar, N., Bayraktar, M., Ibrahim, B., Bozok, T., & Resat, C. M. (2022, October 15). *Evaluation of amino acid profile in serum of patients with covid-19 for providing a new treatment strategy.* Journal of medical biochemistry. https://www.ncbi.nlm.nih.gov/pmc/articles/PMC9618340/

7. Shen, T., & Wang, T. (2021). Metabolic reprogramming in COVID-19. *International Journal of Molecular Sciences, 22*(21), 11475. https://doi.org/10.3390/ijms222111475

8. Bouças, A. P., Rheinheimer, J., & Lagopoulos, J. (2022). Why severe COVID-19 patients are at greater risk of developing depression: A molecular perspective. *The Neuroscientist, 28*(1), 11–19. https://doi.org/10.1177/1073858420967892

9. Chilosi, M., Doglioni, C., Ravaglia, C., Martignoni, G., Salvagno, G. L., Pizzolo, G., Bronte, V., & Poletti, V. (2022). Unbalanced IDO1/IDO2 endothelial expression and skewed kynurenine pathway in the pathogenesis of COVID-19 and post-COVID-19 pneumonia. *Biomedicines, 10*(6), 1332. https://doi.org/10.3390/biomedicines10061332

10. Eroğlu, İ., Eroğlu, B. Ç., & Güven, G. S. (2021). Altered tryptophan absorption and metabolism could underlie long-term symptoms in survivors of coronavirus disease 2019 (COVID-19). *Nutrition, 90*, 111308. https://doi.org/10.1016/j.nut.2021.111308

11. Durante, W. (2023). Glutamine deficiency promotes immune and endothelial cell dysfunction in COVID-19. *International Journal of Molecular Sciences, 24*(8), 7593. https://doi.org/10.3390/ijms24087593

12. Adebayo, A., Varzideh, F., Wilson, S., Gambardella, J., Eacobacci, M., Jankauskas, S. S., Donkor, K., Kansakar, U., Trimarco, V., Mone, P., Lombardi, A., & Santulli, G. (2021). l-Arginine and COVID-19: An update. *Nutrients, 13*(11), 3951. https://doi.org/10.3390/nu13113951

13. Green, S. J. (2020). COVID-19 accelerates endothelial dysfunction and nitric oxide deficiency. *Microbes and Infection, 22*(4–5), 149–150. https://doi.org/10.1016/j.micinf.2020.05.006

14. Wrona, M., & Skrypnik, D. (2022). New-onset diabetes mellitus, hypertension, dyslipidaemia as sequelae of COVID-19 infection—Systematic review. *International Journal of Environmental Research and Public Health, 19*(20), 13280. https://doi.org/10.3390/ijerph192013280

15. Terzic, C. M., & Medina-Inojosa, B. J. (2023). Cardiovascular complications of coronavirus disease-2019. *Physical Medicine and Rehabilitation Clinics of North America, 34*(3), 551–561. https://doi.org/10.1016/j.pmr.2023.03.003

16. Pernas, L. (2021). Cellular metabolism in the defense against microbes. *Journal of Cell Science, 134,* jcs252023. https://doi.org/10.1242/jcs.252023
Low, R. N., Low, R. J., & Akrami, A. (2023). A review of cytokine-based pathophysiology of Long COVID symptoms. *Frontiers in Medicine, 10,* 1011936. https://doi.org/10.3389/fmed.2023.1011936

17. Mohandas, S., Jagannathan, P., Henrich, T. J., Sherif, Z. A., Bime, C., Quinlan, E., Portman, M. A., Gennaro, M., Rehman, J., & RECOVER Mechanistic Pathways Task Force. (2023). Immune mechanisms underlying COVID-19 pathology and post-acute sequelae of SARS-CoV-2 infection (PASC). *eLife, 12,* e86014. https://doi.org/10.7554/eLife.86014

18. Mohandas, S., Jagannathan, P., Henrich, T. J., Sherif, Z. A., Bime, C., Quinlan, E., Portman, M. A., Gennaro, M., Rehman, J., & Force, R. M. P. T. (2023, May 26). *Immune mechanisms underlying COVID-19 pathology and post-acute sequelae of SARS-COV-2 infection (PASC).* eLife. https://elifesciences.org/articles/86014

19. Chen, B., Julg, B., Mohandas, S., Bradfute, S. B., & RECOVER Mechanistic Pathways Task Force. (2023). Viral persistence, reactivation, and mechanisms of long COVID. *eLife, 12,* e86015. https://doi.org/10.7554/eLife.86015

20. Chen, B., Julg, B., Mohandas, S., & Bradfute, S. (2023, May 4). *Viral persistence, reactivation, and mechanisms of long covid.* Recover Mechanistic Pathways Task Force. https://pubmed.ncbi.nlm.nih.gov/37140960/

21. Gold, J. E., Okyay, R. A., Licht, W. E., & Hurley, D. J. (2021). Investigation of Long COVID prevalence and its relationship to Epstein-Barr virus reactivation. *Pathogens, 10*(6), 763. https://doi.org/10.3390/pathogens10060763

22. Henley, S. J., Dowling, N. F., Ahmad, F. B., Ellington, T. D., Wu, M., & Richardson, L. C. (2022). COVID-19 and other underlying causes of cancer deaths — United States, January 2018–July 2022. *MMWR Morbidity and Mortality Weekly Report, 71,* 1583–1588. http://dx.doi.org/10.15585/mmwr.mm7150a3

23. Klein, H. E. (2023, March 22). Kashyap Patel, MD, sees link between COVID-19 and cancer progression, calls for more biomarker testing. *American Journal of Managed Care, Evidence-Based Oncology, 29*(4).

24. Greaves, M. (2018). A causal mechanism for childhood acute lymphoblastic leukaemia. *Nature Reviews Cancer, 18*(8), 471–484. https://doi.org/10.1038/s41568-018-0015-6

25. Dubey, S., Das, S., Ghosh, R., Dubey, M. J., Chakraborty, A. P., Roy, D., Das, G., Dutta, A., Santra, A., Sengupta, S., & Benito-León, J. (2023). The effects of SARS-CoV-2 infection on the cognitive functioning of patients with

pre-existing dementia. *Journal of Alzheimer's Disease Reports, 7*(1), 119–128. https://doi.org/10.3233/ADR-220090

Chapter 8

1. Cardinali, D. P., Brown, G. M., & Pandi-Perumal, S. R. (2022). Possible application of melatonin in long COVID. *Biomolecules, 12*(11), 1646. https://doi.org/10.3390/biom12111646

2. Hsieh, M.-J., Lee, C.-H., Chueh, H.-Y., & Chang, G.-J. (2020). Modulatory effects of BPC 157 on vasomotor tone and the activation of Src-Caveolin-1-endothelial nitric oxide synthase pathway. *Scientific Reports, 10*(1), 17078. https://doi.org/10.1038/s41598-020-74022-y

3. Atieh, O., Daher, J., Durieux, J. C., Abboud, M., Labbato, D., Baissary, J., Koberssy, Z., Ailstock, K., Cummings, M., Funderburg, N. T., & McComsey, G. A. (2025). Vitamins K2 and D3 improve long COVID, fungal translocation, and inflammation: Randomized controlled trial. *Nutrients, 17*(2), 304. https://doi.org/10.3390/nu17020304

4. Coman, A. E., Ceasovschih, A., Petroaie, A. D., Popa, E., Lionte, C., Bologa, C., Haliga, R. E., Cosmescu, A., Slănină, A. M., Bacușcă, A. I., Șorodoc, V., & Șorodoc, L. (2023). The significance of low magnesium levels in COVID-19 patients. *Medicina, 59*(2), 279. https://doi.org/10.3390/medicina59020279

5. Bojadzic, D., Alcazar, O., & Buchwald, P. (2021). Methylene blue inhibits the SARS-CoV-2 spike-ACE2 protein-protein interaction—a mechanism that can contribute to its antiviral activity against COVID-19. *Frontiers in Pharmacology, 11*, 600372. https://doi.org/10.3389/fphar.2020.600372

6. Mazur, A., Maier, J. A. M., Rock, E., Gueux, E., Nowacki, W., & Rayssiguier, Y. (2007). Magnesium and the inflammatory response: potential physiopathological implications. *Archives of Biochemistry and Biophysics, 458*(1), 48–56. https://doi.org/10.1016/j.abb.2006.03.031

7. DiNicolantonio, J. J., & O'Keefe, J. H. (2021). Magnesium and vitamin D deficiency as a potential cause of immune dysfunction, cytokine storm and disseminated intravascular coagulation in COVID-19 patients. *Missouri Medicine, 118*(1), 68–73.

8. Selhub, J., Bagley, L. C., Miller, J., & Rosenberg, I. H. (2000). B vitamins, homocysteine, and neurocognitive function in the elderly. *The American Journal of Clinical Nutrition, 71*(2), 614S–620S. https://doi.org/10.1093/ajcn/71.2.614s

9. Hashemian, H., Qobadighadikolaei, R., Seifnezhad, P., Hassanzadeh Rad, A., Mansouri, S. S., Darini, A., Jamali, F., Rashidpour, F., & Shahrokhi, M. (2017). Efficacy of N-acetylcysteine in children with moderate COVID-19: A placebo-controlled randomized clinical trial. *Nutrients, 9*(12), 1286. https://doi.org/10.3390/nu9121286

10. Lonsdale, D. (2017). *Thiamine deficiency disease, dysautonomia, and high calorie malnutrition.* Catalog - UW-Madison Libraries. https://search.library.wisc.edu/catalog/9912366138702121

11. U.S. Department of Health and Human Services. (2023, February 9). *Office of dietary supplements - thiamin.* NIH Office of Dietary Supplements. https://ods.od.nih.gov/factsheets/Thiamin-HealthProfessional/

12. World Health Organization. (1999, February 23). *Thiamine deficiency and its prevention and control in major emergencies*. World Health Organization. https://www.who.int/publications-detail-redirect/WHO-NHD-99.13

13. Sechi, P. G., & Serra, A. (2007, May). *Wernicke's encephalopathy: New clinical settings and recent advances in diagnosis and management - the lancet neurology*. The Lancet Neurology. https://www.thelancet.com/journals/laneur/article/PIIS1474-4422(07)70104-7/abstract

14. Blitshteyn , S., & Whitelaw, S. (2021, March 30). *Postural orthostatic tachycardia syndrome (POTS) and other autonomic disorders after COVID-19 infection: A case series of 20 patients*. Immunologic research. https://pubmed.ncbi.nlm.nih.gov/33786700/

15. Roger F, B. (2003, December 16). *Thiamin deficiency and brain disorders*. Nutrition research reviews. https://pubmed.ncbi.nlm.nih.gov/19087395/

16. Manzetti, S., Zhang, J., & van der Spoel, D. (2014, January 24). *Thiamin function, metabolism, uptake, and transport | biochemistry*. ACS Publications. https://pubs.acs.org/doi/abs/10.1021/bi401618y

17. Maggini S, Wintergerst ES, Beveridge S, Hornig DH. *Selected vitamins and trace elements support immune function by strengthening epithelial barriers and cellular and humoral immune responses*. (2007). *British Journal of Nutrition*. https://www.cambridge.org/core/journals/british-journal-of-nutrition/article/selected-vitamins-and-trace-elements-

support-immune-function-by-strengthening-epithelial-
barriers-and-cellular-and-humoral-immune-
responses/94B772EB747D1E5CD9FAC8F90937AA9F

18. Costantini, A., Nappo, A., Pala, M. I., & Zappone, A. (2013,
    July 16). *High dose thiamine improves fatigue in multiple
    sclerosis.* BMJ case reports.
    https://pmc.ncbi.nlm.nih.gov/articles/PMC3736110/

19. Wooley, J. A. (2008, October). Review of *Nutrition in
    clinical practice volume 23 number 5. American Society for
    Parenteral and Enteral Nutrition, 23*(5).

20. Otten, J. J., Hellwig, J. P., & Meyers, L. D. (2006, August
    29). *Dietary reference intakes: The essential guide to
    nutrient requirements.* The Essential Guide to Nutrient
    Requirements | The National Academies Press.
    https://nap.nationalacademies.org/catalog/11537/dietary-
    reference-intakes-the-essential-guide-to-nutrient-
    requirements

21. Caly, L., Druce, J. D., Catton, M. G., Jans, D. A., &
    Wagstaff, K. M. (2020). The FDA-approved drug
    ivermectin inhibits the replication of SARS-CoV-2 in vitro.
    Antiviral Research, 178, 104787.
    https://doi.org/10.1016/j.antiviral.2020.104787

22. Zhang, X., Song, Y., Ci, X., An, N., Ju, Y., Li, H., Wang, X.,
    Han, C., Cui, J., & Deng, X. (2008). Ivermectin inhibits
    LPS-induced production of inflammatory cytokines and
    improves LPS-induced survival in mice. *Inflammation,
    57*(11), 524–529. https://doi.org/10.1007/s00011-008-8007-8

23. Mirshahi, F., Aqbi, H. F., Isbell, M., Manjili, S. H., Guo, C.,
    Saneshaw, M., Bandyopadhyay, D., Dozmorov, M., Khosla,
    A., Wack, K., Carrasco-Zevallos, O. M., Idowu, M. O.,

Wang, X.-Y., Sanyal, A. J., & Manjili, M. H. (2022). Distinct hepatic immunological patterns are associated with the progression or inhibition of hepatocellular carcinoma. *Cell Reports, 38*(9), 110454. https://doi.org/10.1016/j.celrep.2022.110454

24. Vottero, P., Tavernini, S., Santin, A. D., Scheim, D. E., Tuszynski, J. A., & Aminpour, M. (2023). Computational prediction of the interaction of ivermectin with fibrinogen. *International Journal of Molecular Sciences, 24*(14), 11449. https://doi.org/10.3390/ijms241411449

25. Fahmy, M.-E. A., Shalaby, M. A., Issa, R., Badawi, M., Magdy, M., Afife, A. A., & Abdel-Aal, A. A. (2023). Ivermectin modulated cerebral γ-aminobutyric acid (GABA) and reduced the number of chronic *Toxoplasma gondii* cysts significantly in the brains of immunocompromised mice. *Journal of Parasitic Diseases, 47*(3), 635–643. https://doi.org/10.1007/s12639-023-01608-4

26. de Melo Júnior, E. J. M., Raposo, M. J., Lisboa Neto, J. A., Diniz, M. F. A., Marcelino Júnior, C. A. C., & Sant'Ana, A. E. G. (2002). Medicinal plants in the healing of dry socket in rats: microbiological and microscopic analysis. *Phytomedicine, 9*(2), 109-116. https://doi.org/10.1078/0944-7113-00087

27. Zilberman-Itskovich, S., Catalogna, M., Sasson, E., Elman-Shina, K., Hadanny, A., Lang, E., Finci, S., Polak, N., Fishlev, G., Korin, C., Shorer, R., Parag, Y., Sova, M., & Efrati, S. (2022). Hyperbaric oxygen therapy improves neurocognitive functions and symptoms of post-COVID condition: randomized controlled trial. *Scientific Reports, 12*(1), 11252. https://doi.org/10.1038/s41598-022-15565-0

28. Silberstein, S. D., Yuan, H., Najib, U., Ailani, J., Lopes de Morais, A., Mathew, P. G., Liebler, E., Tassorelli, C., & Diener, H.-C. (2020). Non-invasive vagus nerve stimulation for primary headache: A clinical update. *Cephalalgia*, 40(12), 1370–1384. https://doi.org/10.1177/0333102420941864

29. Riley, D., Hao, J. J., Kiene, H., Kienle, G., Mittelman, M., & Plotnikoff, G. A. (2012). Global advances in health and medicine. *Global Advances in Health and Medicine*, 1(1), 5–7. https://doi.org/10.7453/gahmj.2012.1.1.001

30. Brossier, D. W., Tume, L. N., Briant, A. R., Jotterand Chaparro, C., Moullet, C., Rooze, S., Verbruggen, S. C. A. T., Marino, L. V., Alsohime, F., Beldjilali, S., Chiusolo, F., Costa, L., Didier, C., Ilia, S., Joram, N. L., Kneyber, M. C. J., Kühlwein, E., Lopez, J., López-Herce, J., Mayberry, H. F., Mehmeti, F., Mierzewska-Schmidt, M., Miñambres Rodríguez, M., Morice, C., Pappachan, J. V., Porcheret, F., Reis Boto, L., Schlapbach, L. J., Tekguc, H., Tziouvas, K., Parienti, J.-J., Goyer, I., & Valla, F. V. (2022). ESPNIC clinical practice guidelines: intravenous maintenance fluid therapy in acute and critically ill children—a systematic review and meta-analysis. *Intensive Care Medicine*, 48(12), 1691–1708. https://doi.org/10.1007/s00134-022-06882-z

31. Şahan, E., Şahan, S., & Karamanlıoğlu, M. (2015). Respiratory physiology & neurobiology. *Respiratory Physiology & Neurobiology*, 208, 57. https://doi.org/10.1016/j.resp.2014.10.003

32. Guo, K., Lu, Y., Wang, X., Duan, Y., Li, H., Gao, F., & Wang, J. (2024, September 23). *Multi-level exploration of auricular acupuncture: From traditional Chinese medicine*

theory to modern medical application. Frontiers in neuroscience. https://pmc.ncbi.nlm.nih.gov/articles/PMC11456840/#:~:text=Relevant%20studies%20have%20demonstrated%20that,direction%20for%20personalized%20treatment%20plans.

www.ingramcontent.com/pod-product-compliance
Lightning Source LLC
Chambersburg PA
CBHW071502140726
47997CB00005B/1820